Broken Hearts and Empty Chairs

One Woman's Journey

Heart Attack >> Integrative Care >> Recovery

Pam Papas

Broken Hearts and Empty Chairs
One Woman's Journey

Heart Attack, Alternative Care, Recovery

Papas Press LLC. Visit us at -www.papaspress.com

Contact Author-emptychairs7@aol.com

Cover design by: Kimberly Martin, www.self-pub.net

Other books by Pam Papas:

New Normals Reclaiming a Life of Significance

Disclaimer

This is not a medical book. It is not intended to replace the advice of your doctor. The information provided in this book should not be construed as personal medical advice or instruction. No action should be taken based solely on the contents of this book. Readers should consult appropriate health professionals on any matter relating to their health and well being. The information and opinions provided here are believed to be accurate and sound, based on the best judgment available to the author, but readers who fail to consult appropriate health authorities assume the risk of any injuries. This book is not responsible for errors or omissions. Before you attempt any exercise routine or therapy it should be preapproved by your doctor or therapist. Each illness is different and each person's capacity to heal varies as well. As a result there is no "one size fits all" treatment plan or pathway to healing. This book offers suggestions based on the positive results I experienced during my recovery process.

About Me

I was born in Chicago in the early 1950's to parents that survived The Great Depression, and World War II. We were a large, middle class family, typical of the Baby Boom Generation. I grew up surrounded by folks with an impeccable work ethic. They were proud, humble; salt of the earth types, of Polish descent. There was so much to learn from all the busy hands. Nothing was wasted; everyone had a pot of soup simmering on the stove. Everything was hand washed, from dishes to floors. It was a contradiction of time; less complicated yet more difficult.

We had a Rosary in lieu of jewelry, and a prayer book, instead of a book collection. It was a time when pennies were still valuable. They went in the collection basket at Sunday Mass or for a special treat; penny candy.

No one took vacations, but Lake Michigan beaches were within a long walking distance. Hot summer nights we all slept on the back porch hoping for a breeze to sneak through the brick metropolis. We were introduced to star gazing, and encouraged to wish upon the stars. Oh… and there's no cold like, Chicago cold. Big families knew the key to warmth; five kids snuggled in one twin bed. This modest existence was a privilege, as it defined my life path of faith, family, hard work, and hope.

As a young girl, my day-dreams were filled with being a Mom. Other young girls were already aspiring to be teachers, nurses and secretaries; the field of opportunity wasn't huge. Although none of those other careers interested me, I did say that I thought I would like to manage a business one day. That was the cause of some raised eyebrows.

Who knew I was prophesying at such a young age. For all of my dreams came true. I've enjoyed a thirty year relationship with my husband, Chris. We have five wonderful, grown children and have been blessed to date with eight extraordinary grandchildren. I had the benefit of a long and satisfying career in Hospitality. It spans over thirty years with various management positions in the Hotel and Restaurant Industries.

Today, I'm the President of New Normals and Papas Press LLC. I have found purpose through personal pain, and the pain of others. I'm an activist for survivors of stroke/brain injury, a voice for caregivers, and an advocate for women with heart disease. We currently reside in Pennsylvania near all of our children and grandchildren.

Dedication, Acknowledgement, In Memory

My life and this book are dedicated to The Glory of God...

To Brian, my son, when you listened to your heart you saved mine...

For my husband, children, and grandchildren, your energy called me home...

In memory of my sister, Kim- Always...

For Mom, my first love...

Contents

Preface:

I found it impossible to tell my story without my cast of characters, my family. However, I would need to add a glossary for all of their names alone, especially if I added in-laws. Instead I refer to them in relationship; daughter, grandson, etc. rather than their proper names. There are some exceptions, which were necessary to the conversation. Here is a snap shot into our life as it relates to the book.

One of my great joys is our gathering for Sunday dinners. In recent years our immediate family has grown from our original seven to twenty members. When we're together, we celebrate life; from birth through each birthday, from report cards to promotions. We welcome our informal flock with love, and an abundance of freshly prepared foods. Our kids bring it all home; their hopes, dreams, problems, children, friends, new pets and yes, even some laundry.

My grandson once wrote a report for his English class that best describes us; the topic was, "Family Celebrations." He shared his recipe on how to make the best ice cream sundae ever. "You need a huge bowl," he said, "and five cousins; two, to scoop the ice cream, one, pours the toppings, we all squirt the whip cream"… you get the picture. Then he declared himself a really lucky kid because he had such a great family. He makes my heart smile. That report held center stage on the refrigerator for at least a year.

While we celebrate life, we also remember our dead. Many years later we may still mark your day by preparing your favorite meal. Dad's favorite was spareribs and sauerkraut; heavy on the caraway seeds. Mom passed just last year. She enjoyed a freshly baked, end piece of crusty bread, and she loved to shop. So for *her* we went to the bakery, before we shopped. These purely symbolic gestures provide comfort to the living, and sustenance to the spirit. Possibly one of your greatest achievements is to leave a legacy of fond memories, and let it be said-"She lived a good life. It was just her time."

Perhaps you would say my family accepts, with reverence, the circle of life. However, it's been our experience, when that circle is broken too young or without warning, the suffering is far worse than in a natural death. The shock and trauma of the loss may repeat itself each year, in its season, for some time to come. Solely because you're robbed of the opportunity to say goodbye, you search for that peace in closure. We want solace for those we love, even in death. Unfortunately sudden deaths don't allow it. You'll mark these days as well, probably different. Maybe you'll attend your place of worship and light a candle. Sit vigil at a cemetery. Or in a desperate attempt to have a living memorial maybe you'll plant their favorite tree or flower... I have a garden full of Lilies... Until we meet again.

Large families can be wonderful. There's more joy to celebrate but, unfortunatley by sheer numbers they're more vunerable to heartaches as well. I think that phrase soul mates is over used and often misused, but I believe we have soul ties. There are people we were meant to spend our lives with. The true test of a soul mate is someone that accepts their support role through all of life's traumas. For our family, the journey has united us. We are stronger individually and collectively because of it.

"To whom much is given much is required" —*Luke 12:48*

Introduction

"Above all else guard your heart, for it is the wellspring of life."
—Proverbs 23:7

For many years now, I've tried to draw attention to my special day. It was by the Grace of God that I survived a heart attack and sudden death. However, for some reason when I say to my family, "Hey Guys, it's May 23rd and I'm here… another year." Their mood and response is a rather subdued. "Oh… that's great Mom." My presumption is no one wants to be reminded of how fragile life is. They're usually very supportive of my attempts to make the best of life's moments, except on this day. In my "Glory" I want to sing and dance to- "Twist and Shout," and savor each bite of my annual cheeseburger. They want to forget. I suppose it's like my Lily garden; there are anniversaries that are sovereign to our soul only.

This year I achieved my ten year anniversary. I was feeling a deep sense of gratitude as I marked the day with a thank you letter to my Cardiologist. He managed my heart care for a couple of years after my heart attack. Though it had been many years since we had any contact, I was confident as patients go, I'd be pretty hard to forget. For almost a year I had one complication after the other. A renewed respect and gratitude for his meticulous care was unleashed when my memories collided with the current female heart disease information.

5

It was during one of those, *Heart Awareness Campaigns*. The morning news programs communicated these awful facts. I listened carefully with sadness and anger to the unfortunate statistics of female mortality after a heart attack. Their information must be faulty I thought, surely we progressed in the ten years. But changing the channel didn't work. The statistics and percentages were about the same network to network. There was no good news, except for the fact that I was alive and well. Somehow I managed this storm of unknowns. And recognized my care was probably superior to most, as I signed my letter: *With a grateful heart*, Pam.

Depending on what report you read the statistics differ slightly, but they're not declining. Approximately 42% of women die within a year of a heart attack in the United States according to The National Women's Health Information Center, CDC. How can this be? Worldwide, 8.6 million women will die from heart diseases this year, 435,000 American women will have heart attacks this year and 267,000 women will die from those heart attacks. Under the age of fifty, female heart attacks are twice as likely as male, to be fatal. It is the number one killer of women. Annually, it kills more women than all the cancers combined. Yet 60% of women still believe the leading cause of death among them is cancer. (Women Heart Foundation)

Unfortunately, 70% of women will have early warning signs with sudden onset of extreme weakness that too many us, ignore. Why do we ignore it? My belief is we have taught ourselves how to overcome, or compensate for our exhaustion. Let's face it; too many of us continue to do a lousy job of making ourselves a priority.

Are we asking the right questions? What component are we missing when some live through the trauma of the heart attack, but still die within the year? Was the proper support system in place for a complete recovery? Why did I and so many others survive the heart attack, while many women die instantly? Are there any common denominators? Is it possible that at onset of the heart attack, the survivor group all took two aspirins? If so, let's scream it from the rooftops!

Education and advocacy efforts are more difficult with a heart disease. I believe it's because it's silent. With a shower and a little makeup forty eight hours after the heart attack, on the surface, I appeared fine. We don't lose our hair. Generally our external body isn't altered in any way; most damage is internal and not obvious to the eye. I'm very sensitive to the plight of the survivors of cancer. Someone very dear to me recently went through a horrific year with cancer. My belief is, because it attacks our female vanity we tend to pay more attention to it.

Maybe a heart campaign designed to highlight the 267,000 empty chairs. A true representation of the astronomical loss of life, just last year alone, would be more effective. Those chairs once held our mothers, daughters, grandmothers, sisters, and our friends...If it hasn't already, it will surely affect you in this lifetime. It has exceeded epidemic proportions.

It is also my belief that many of us feel we somehow caused our heart disease. In fact we've been told so. This notion that heart disease is completely preventable is not true. In many cases and until your cardiologist orders you to have a complete blood panel I wouldn't be so ready to accept this thinking. Indeed we should all follow healthy life style guidelines, but having said that, as I have become a student of heart disease I've seen too many people die unaware of inherited factors. Rule out the inherited factors before you accept the responsibility of "doing it wrong," because simply life style change, may not improve your outcome.

It's more common than you think for a jogger or marathon runner to suddenly die of a heart attack. How do we explain this; perfect weight, body mass index, always embraced a healthy life style. What do we tell their loved ones? What should they have done differently? If we want to prevent more untimely losses from heart disease the medical community needs to standardize the tests that predict a complete picture of our coronary risk factors. It is a panel of blood test much like the normal cholesterol test, but unlike cholesterol test, they predict toxic genetic factors and in some cases, the early onset of heart disease. The tests are called: VAP test or Spectracell test.

When we discover the truth, the real deal, behind our disease, we can take the appropriate measures to combat it. How many women died this year feeling confused or guilty for not having done enough to prevent their illness? That's just wrong. Too many of us already operate from a baseline of guilt, let's just heap it on.

We will probably never know the psychological state of the women that died within a year of a heart attack; and unfortunately I would also suspect that most died without complete blood testing. Having survived that first year with numerous complications, there is much to be learned from my experience.

One day, we will find a cure for heart disease. However, and in the meantime, I believe with proper, complete blood testing we can save lives by preventing heart attacks. You cannot address the inherited cause if you're not aware of its existence. You can have heart disease without having a heart attack.

Cardiologists have also identified a temporary heart condition that can cause a heart attack. It's brought on by a surge of stress hormones, accompanied by stressful situations; a sudden break up of a long marriage or a death of a loved one. This "Broken Heart Syndrome," is the result of a devastating life event. There's yet so much to be learned about the female heart and its tie to our emotions.

The thought of this book originated ten years ago when my life was threatened by heart disease. Today my inspiration is simply those empty chairs. While I survived, our family has also endured the impact of that empty chair. My call to action came when I was reminded of the unacceptable loss of life that first year after a heart attack. When I narrowed my focus of information to the two years' post heart attack, the book suddenly came alive with purpose. It was time.

That's where I focused my efforts. I'll walk you through the strategies I incorporated into my healing process. And the road I took to get there. I resurrected memories from a painful time in my life to be able to say to you, "I remember well. You are not alone. We give completely, that's our purpose, our rite of passage. We are nurturers. We were physically overdrawn and finally, we broke." Women impacted by disease, whether heart disease or cancer, share many of the same secrets and feelings. We ignored our soul whispers for self care, and some had too many traumatic yesterdays.

How we choose to move through life now will define our future. I hope each of my stories inspires your confidence and encourages your own advocacy. I share my knowledge and experience of Alternative/Holistic healing approaches. This is most important, as you select and build your own support system. Like so many diseases there is not a "one size fits all" cure. There is hope and options are available to achieve wholeness. Our symptoms vary, as well as the level of needed care.

Before I could put my pen to the paper I needed something more measurable. I'd been in search of a happy ending. The ten year anniversary was my turning point; I'm here. I also understood that I had to walk through it completely, to help others, and to find peace on the other side. There is not an X-ray that can provide me with a spirit of wellness. In spite of the medical diagnosis or prognosis, I had to pronounce myself "healed" in my heart and soul. Once you're diagnosed with heart disease or cancer, the label never disappears. It's a life long association with that disease; you are a survivor of… or a heart patient.

For this purpose I have re-examined my survival experience and know it was dependent on addressing more than my physical heart. I am grateful for Conventional Medicine and believe in its importance. It saved my life. However, it was an Integrative approach; a combination of Conventional and Holistic/Alternative efforts that fueled my healing. The wisdom I gained in the transition taught me how to protect and heal my spiritual heart.

Had I remained on course with only the Conventional Medical approaches, surely my life would have slipped into the category of: The women that die within a year of a heart attack. Because you see, I followed all the guidelines, did exactly what I was told to do, and during that first year, I often thought I was dying too.

Chapter 1:
Surrender

"I postpone death by living, by suffering, by error, by risking,
by giving, by losing." —Helen Keller

The year was 2000; it was a beautiful May morning. The sunlight danced in between our bedroom window blinds, as the gentle breeze moved the blinds in perfect sequence back and forth. Each breeze carried the glorious scent of spring's peonies and you could hear the first sounds of baby robins as they rose from slumber in search of food. Ahh… and finally I wake to capture the aroma of good, strong coffee filling the air. It was time to get up.

There was no need for an alarm clock; three of our five kids and our granddaughter were still living at home. I'd stay out of the line of fire while they'd try to cram what would take the average person a half hour to do, into fifteen minutes. "Yep," I'd smile to myself, "They're all efficiency experts." I listened as they hurried through their morning rituals; preparing for work, college, and high school. All of them rushing; doors opening, door closing, the jingling of keys. The morning was complete with a meltdown as our daughter negotiated with her two year old daughter. With desperation in her voice, "Mommy will tape it… I promise… you won't miss it. We'll watch it together when we come home." "But…" my granddaughter insisted,

"I don't want to go to college today Mommy...I just want to watch Barney!" (Her day care was at the university her mom attended.) I knew it was safe to come out of my bedroom when I heard the third "Bye Mom."

Waking up to all this commotion, for me, was the perfect setting. This was my life. I honestly never tired from hearing their activity. I am a grateful woman and I know I've been blessed. This morning scenario would typically stimulate happy emotions or at least encourage a smile. However, not that morning, I woke overwhelmed with a frightening feeling of doom.

While my husband, Chris, dressed and packed for a business trip; I tried to describe this feeling to him. "Something's wrong," I said. "Maybe you shouldn't go."My husband always said that I operated from a sixth sense that he didn't have and it confused him. On this day I wish he would have listened to it. Once we established that "I" personally didn't feel sick, he suggested that maybe I had a bad dream or something. He left for the airport with the promise that he could be home in a couple of hours if he was needed.

The feeling of impending doom accompanied me as I dragged myself out of bed and eventually to work. I felt weak and shaky. I had a slight ache in my left arm and shoulder. I told myself, "I must have slept on it wrong." I remember that after eating lunch I felt worse. So now I had impending doom, I'm weak, achy, and shaky with stomach pains. I had plans after work to meet my daughters-in-law to purchase christening outfits for my grandsons' dual baptism. No aches and pains were keeping me away.

On my way to meet them I had a near miss car accident with two semi trucks. Somehow I found myself between two trucks on a two lane highway. It's a miracle in itself that I'm here to tell this story. There was not a scratch on me or the car, but maybe something worse happened in that moment, because as I tensed up moving through the trucks I felt upper body tightness and a tingling sensation in my arms. My heart was pounding, as was my head, but after a few minutes I told myself that I pulled a muscle.

When I arrived the kids were waiting for me. We were all excited to see each other. As I told my daughters-in-law about the truck ordeal and reached to pick up my infant grandson, I started to sweat profusely and felt a sharp pain in my back. I suggested we sit down for a few minutes. When they handed me a glass of water I instinctively reached for my purse and took a couple of aspirins. A few minutes later we tried shopping again, and I just didn't feel well. I excused myself with apologies and drove past the hospital on the way home. I did have a brief thought of stopping and just as quickly talked myself out of it, "No I'm fine."

When I got home my daughters were waiting for me as they had already received a call from my daughters-in-law that I was not well, and in route. It was unusual for me to be sick; I thought I was a healthy forty-six years old. I caught maybe one cold a year. After I warded off all the, "let's call Dad... let's go to the hospital," suggestions, my son Brian walked in the door. He was supposed to have a softball game nearby, but it was suddenly cancelled, so he decided to stop by to say, "Hi."

His younger sisters immediately accosted him with the details of my day's events. He listened carefully as they complained, "And she won't even let us call Dad." Now, Brian started with questions, "How do you feel Mom?" "I feel like I pulled a muscle in my chest, I'm just slightly uncomfortable not really in pain," I said. "Get your purse Mom we're going to the hospital," he commanded, "We'll just get an x-ray and you'll be home in an hour." "But Brian I really don't think"… "Let's go Mom!" he insisted, "You're getting this checked out. I'm not leaving you until you do."

My Brian is a no nonsense type, who obviously knew how to handle me. He listened well; he could have been my echo. Raising five kids was not an easy task and at times I found it easier to say, "Cut the crap just do it," rather than entertaining more unwarranted conversation.

Though my symptoms were vague and disorganized throughout the day, when you combined them they weren't painting a particularly good picture; feeling of doom, upset stomach, ache in my left arm, tingling in both arms, profuse sweating, tightness in my chest…So back to the hospital I had just passed thirty minutes before…

After surrendering to the idea, it was a quiet car ride between us. In the stillness I started to experience yet another symptom; I had a mild pain radiating in my jaw. This was the one symptom of a heart attack that I knew. There was no way for me to try to interpret it as anything else. I slid into a trance of silent prayer.

As we got closer to the hospital I took prayer to a new level and started negotiating with God, "Look this is not possible two of our grandsons will be baptized next week and our daughter's high school graduation is the following week. God, are you sure I need to go through this? Is there any way out?"But as I felt the pain radiate my jaw I realized my schedule of upcoming events wasn't His concern. I've tried fighting with God before; my arms just aren't long enough. As we entered the hospital parking lot I surrendered again and said, "Please God, just stay with me."

Fortunately for me our community hospital was more advanced in their heart knowledge than most hospitals around the country. Other hospitals were still sending women home without an EKG, and with an acid reducer for their discomfort. This was ten years ago. Until someone started counting, they thought this was a "man's disease."

As they wheeled me in to one of the emergency room cubicles with the nurse attending to me, my son left to register me. As he drew the curtain between us he said, "I'll see you in a few minutes Mom, are you sure you don't want me to call Dad?" "I'm sure; it's just a pulled muscle. Why worry him. Relax Brian, I'll be here when you get back," I joked.

The nurse took my vitals and then instructed me to put on the hospital gown. She commented that I looked too young to have a son as old as Brian. I loved her immediately. "I have four grandchildren," I proudly announced, "and five children." We shared middle age mom stories, and a couple of laughs, when she asked me to lie down so she could connect me to the EKG monitor. That's all I remember. As I did, I went into cardiac arrest.

Brian remembers hearing the "Code Blue" emergency call over the speaker system just moments after leaving me. He didn't even make it to the registration area yet, but quickly justified in his mind that it wasn't for me-"No way," he thought, "She was just sitting up and laughing, no way." While Brian was searching my wallet for my insurance cards I was receiving my first electrical jolt to restart my heart. They administered all three possible electrical shocks to my heart before I came back.

Was there a bright light, a tunnel, a feeling of serenity, or deep sense of peace, so often described? No, I felt none of that. I do have a recollection of a hallway. In my vision it was a typical hospital corridor complete with lots of activity. I didn't see the activity; I felt it, a pure energy. I could hear scrambled, soft spoken female voices. While I have no memory of exactly what was said to me, I do feel their gentle spirits were quickly trying to guide me back, it was not my time.

Leaning over me as I regained consciousness; his starched white coat brushed my arm. I tried to read his name tag to no avail, just a blurry maze of letters, but clearly ending in M.D. This young, handsome doctor, just inches from my face and speaking loudly, said to me, "Mrs. Papas can you hear me?" As I opened my eyes I must have nodded as he said, "Mrs. Papas do you know your husband's full *Greek* name…his *Greek* name," he repeated. With his emphasis on the word Greek I understood and tried to respond, when I realized I had an oxygen mask covering most of my face. It felt so hot and uncomfortable, I tried to pull it off when many hands came flying towards me explaining; "Oh no Honey," someone said, "You need that." As they held it slightly away from my face I replied, "Yes… his Greek name is Papanastasiou… Christos Papanastasiou." With my response the ER Doctor proclaimed, "She's back! We got her! She made it!" When they started to cheer I heard their excitement and felt their joy, but didn't really comprehend why, or what was truly happening. This talented group had just brought me back from death.

Once they rather cleverly assessed my mental state with the Papas test, and established all of me came back, (by the way the ER Doc was Greek with a very long name) I heard him outside the curtain updating my son. "We lost your Mom for a bit." With that Brian immediately interrupted him and in an abrupt tone, "What do you mean you lost her, I just left her with you. How could you lose her?" "No son, that was a poor choice of words on my part," calmly, the doctor replied. "Your mom suffered a heart attack and we were able to bring her back. She was clinically dead for a short while. The Cardiologist is with her now, and he will administer a clot busting drug." Brian's voice went from anger to deep sadness in a blink and a tear when he said, "Can I see her?" "For a few minutes," he warned, "we need her to rest." I suddenly realized I was naked and began to cry, "Please don't let my son in until you cover me." Now under the supervision of the Cardiologist, he sternly warned me to calm down as he instructed that blankets be carefully placed over me, around the monitors, wires and tubes.

I'll probably never know the extent of memories burned into Brian's sub-conscious as he re-entered the room. I was relieved to have a blanket, didn't think to ask for a mirror and as crazy as this sounds, I remember wiping under my eyes, worried that my mascara had run. How ridiculous, I just died and I'm worried about how I might look. What does someone look like moments after a death experience, maybe older or wiser? Did I glow? It's certainly easier to laugh at myself ten years later.

The conversation between us was short. He was obviously upset. He came in long enough to say, "I'm calling Dad," and I simply said, "I'm so sorry Brian... Be careful how you tell your sisters and brothers, I want everyone safe." What a burden to be saddled with. One by one our kids appeared at my bedside that night. I felt their anguish. I would have liked nothing more than to wave a magic wand and heal all their fears. However for the first time in their lives it was all about me. And whatever energy I had left at that moment, I needed it to survive. For me, being the center of attention was as foreign as the heart attack. I truly despised having my family hovering over me, it made me more determined to fight and go home.

My husband was able to catch the last flight out of Chicago to Baltimore. If he were one minute later he would not have been able to keep his morning promise that he could be "home in a couple of hours" if he was needed. At some point I woke to find him sitting at my bedside. I apologized to him too for being sick. He tried to console me, and I cried myself back to sleep.

The next day I was transported by ambulance to a larger Baltimore hospital's Cardiac Catherization Lab. It would be determined if I needed an angioplasty procedure and/or a stent. My kids had already

20

done their homework and found out that the Cardiologist assigned to me was the head of the Lab. He performs over three hundred of these procedures yearly. "He's the best, Mom. He's the man!" My sons assured me.

When they wheeled me in to the Cardiac Catherization Lab, I was greeted by the man my kids investigated, the Interventional Cardiologist. I connected with him immediately. He held my hand and told me I was, "Too young to be so sick." My response was, "Death is not an option. I have too much yet to do." He told me we were the same age and he understood. He promised me he wouldn't let anything happen to me, and that I was going to be okay. Looking back that was quite a profound thirty second conversation. I don't remember being terribly anxious about the procedure. Maybe due in part to the medications I was on. I did feel safe in his care.

When I reflect on my behavior, the utter state of denial I was in prior to, and during the day of, the heart attack I'm able to recognize it was born literally from a trusted source. I'll need to take you back in time to explain…

Notes from my heart:

What I know for sure, ten years later: There is probably no greater moment of truth than those crucial moments before your physical body faces death. I surrendered my health to God, but not my life. I pleaded for more time. I instinctively knew to visualize my future. I took reign of my mind/soul. With a divine determination, I sought, and then expected, a miracle.

1. Male and female heart attack symptoms are generally very different. Female symptoms are often more subtle.

2. Listen to your intuitions, sixth senses that gut feeling.

3. The feeling of doom I experienced that day; it's often reported as a symptom.

4. Men may experience crushing chest pain while women may just feel a slight tightness, like a bra that's too tight.

5. Women's symptoms range from mild stomach ache to nausea. Women often experience extreme tiredness and shortness of breath.

6. One might experience tightness or ache in the left arm. I had both, plus a tingling sensation that radiated through both arms.

7. An ache or pain radiating in the jaw line

8. If you suspect your having a heart attack studies have shown taking aspirin may improve your outcome.

9. My heart attack was ten years ago. The emergency care I received was very much the exception. Not the rule. I have heard recent stories of emergency rooms not reacting to these symptoms, for both males and females. Make sure you insist on an EKG and blood work to test for troponin levels before you leave the emergency room.

10. If you find yourself needing an angioplasty or stent there is a specialty in Cardiology; an Interventional Cardiologist. Generally, they have performed more of these procedures than the average Cardiologist and provide improved outcomes for their patients as they have perfected their technique.

11. Its common after a heart attack to be fearful. There's fear of another heart attack and of sudden death. You may need to seek professional help.

12. After a heart attack your emotions can be in great conflict. You're very grateful for another chance at life and confused about the depression you may feel. You may need to seek help for this as well.

Chapter 2:
The Anomaly

"Faith is the strength by which a shattered world shall emerge into the light." —Leo Buscaglia

In my treasure chest of memories I hold dear you'll find my best day ever, my favorite gift… However for twelve years and running, the winner of the, "Best gift I ever gave," was in 1998. It was for my younger sister, Kim. On March 31st she was celebrating her 41st birthday. We always made a big fuss on the milestone birthdays 21, 30, 40 etc. The other regular birthdays were celebrated with maybe a small gift, surely a card, and of course a phone call. But, this was an odd year, number 41. The spirit just moved me. When I heard her reaction I was so glad it did. She called that day to say, "You sent me flowers!" There was surprise and happiness in her voice. She giggled as she told me how flowers received at her house were usually for her neighbors that worked all day, as she described the spring bouquet I sent her. "It's just perfect," she went on, "There's every color flower you can imagine. Maybe as these dry I'll try to replace them with a silk version. Really Pam they're that pretty. I love all the bright colors in my kitchen. They look great."

We were all born in Chicago and later grew up in a working class, Chicago suburb. A family of five kids; I was three years older than

Kim. Our brother was born between us, just eleven months younger than me. We are complete with two older sisters. In Chicago they have a name for siblings born within a year, they're referred to as "Irish Twins!" They were common among the Catholic families, but you didn't have to be Irish, just Catholic. We are Polish, and there were plenty of jokes about that as well.

Kim was the baby in the family. She was always a natural beauty. However, she was rather shy and definitely territorial. No one became her friend easily. Even new family members like our spouses had to earn their way into her good grace. Once she let you in, you were a lifer.

Growing up we always shared the same bedroom. I taught her how to read. She was my fashion consultant. After we left home we shared an apartment for awhile. I kept all her secrets, she kept mine. On the surface she appeared to be strong and overly protective of all of us, much like our Dad.

However, I always held her close. Because somehow I knew, that truly she was the fragile one.

Like most Chicagoans she was a lifetime resident. Few people born there ever leave. We moved away a year after she got married, I was about thirty years old at the time. She was furious with me for going. She never let me forget how she was there to help with my kids and I wasn't going to be there for her, and her kids. With all her disapproval, she was my first visitor when we moved, and I made it home as often as I could.

My husband's career uprooted us from the Midwest to the East Coast; we lived in Maryland at the time. Like clockwork I would call at least once a week. It was during a phone call a few days earlier, I started to worry. Kim sounded exhausted, almost breathless. We were raised to be tough stock, not "complainers" and as a result we learned to be good listeners. Her life was not easy. While I was able to justify her tiredness, her voice frightened me. She had three young children, one child had serious disabilities, and her husband worked long hours. She too worked a part-time job. Although she enjoyed the help and companionship of our Mom, Kim's voice set me on high alert.

When she called about the flowers, I was prepared. I encouraged her to come for a vacation. "My treat, bring Mom, we have plenty of hands at my house to help with the kids. We'll take a tour through Washington DC and a couple of days to relax at the ocean. Come on Kim, Chicago winters are just too long. Let's take a break." That was our plan for June, just around the corner. Her voice brightened as we planned our trip.

On April 29, 1998 I woke up crying. This had never happened to me before. I was frantic trying to understand what was wrong. What did I do yesterday? Why am I crying? I felt so incredibly sad. I tried to remember. But, nothing jumped out at me. I got up, checked on the kids and made excuses to call our older kids. I called my husband. He was traveling that week. Everybody was fine. Once I was able to stop crying, I got dressed and went to work. What a horrible way to start the day. I knew in my soul something was wrong.

If Kim had just turned forty-one, both born March babies, I was forty-four at the time. Our family had already lived through more than our share of tragedies, or so I thought. Most days I had an ongoing dialog with God as I fought to understand and stay in faith. *"Please God guide and protect my family."* Sadness hung over me like a cruel cloud all day.

The waking up in tears and reality came together that evening when the phone rang. My daughter said, "Mom… its Uncle Tommy." As she reached to hand me the phone, my first thought was; "Oh my God no, something is wrong. He never calls at night. It must be about Mom. My heart was pounding as I said, "Hi Tommy." His voice cracked when he tried to speak. "Kim's… gone… Pam… they think it was heart attack… I'm at the emergency room with Mom… they tried to bring Kim back…they did all they could…She's gone… Before I went into a state of complete hysteria I think I made him repeat it again before I started screaming and handed the phone to my daughter. I remember and can feel the pain in those screams to this day as I pleaded; Oh God no… please God no… her children, our Mom… I sobbed and screamed for hours.

My husband tried to get a flight home but couldn't. Instead he tried to calm me down over the phone, which was not his best idea. That night I was unable to control myself. I needed to yell and scream and cry… my heart was breaking. I tried to explain to our kids sometime later it was as though Kim was being ripped from my soul. For hours on end I continued to walk in circles from our living room, foyer, dining room, kitchen, family room and then I repeated the circle over and over and over again. Eventually all five of our kids came home that night.

Under my husband's direction, my son's encouraged me to drink a little wine that they had laced with sleeping pills. It took a lot to penetrate that pain. But finally my circles became slower and confused, and they were able to walk me upstairs to my bed.

By now it was well past midnight. As I sat defiantly on the edge of my bed softly weeping, I thought I heard birds outside my window. When I asked my kids, "Does anyone else hear these birds?" They all responded in unison, "Yes!" "Mom the birds are really here, we all hear them too. They have been singing for hours now." Were they birds? Were they Angels? Birds' singing in the middle of the night was sign enough for me that the hand of God was upon us.

I listened to the choir of birds as they serenaded us, with a harmony of a heart wrenching opera. This was not a cheerful sound; no, they were grieving with us. Their musical rendition pierced my soul. Never have I heard such a sound. I have no doubt they were sent to comfort us. Glory to God…

Our home had an in-law suite that was always in use by our kids. One by one, it was a revolving door as my husband and I set a rule that you can only occupy it for a one year period. It helped all of our kids to get a good start; save for a house, clear up past mistakes (credit card debt) or a place to heal a broken wing.

Our present occupants were my eldest son and his family. When I woke to feel my four year old grandson crawling into bed with me the next morning, I was sickened at the thought that he heard me the night before. Is it possible that he slept through it? Lying still in bed pretending to be asleep, I felt him cuddle next to me under the blankets. He then very carefully reached for the remote to turn on his morning cartoon line-up. I could feel my swollen eyes. I knew I had to get up. I had so much to do. I dreaded the thought of that day.

It wasn't long before they realized my grandson was missing and the cavalry came and tried to lure him out of my bed with sign language. I could feel him confidently shake his head "No" and move in closer to me. They would wave and whisper, "Come here!" and he would "shush" them, and whisper, "Nana's sleeping." One frustrated parent would leave and the next one would try, finally they gave up.

But my little protector held watch over me and what he thought was my sleeping body. As I laid there and recalled my brother's words the night before, "Kim's gone," my tears though now silent, began again. After a few minutes I felt my grandson's precious finger tips on my face, as he wiped away my tears, he whispered, "You know Nana, the Angels came last night and they cried with you." "I know Honey," I said, "Wasn't that so nice of them to come?" "Yes it was," he continued. "Daddy said they're your Angels…Nana's Angels?" "Well he's almost right, they are all of our Angels, they came for all of us," I continued, "Now…how about you go downstairs and ask your Dad to bring me a cup of coffee. I have a little bit of a headache." Like a flash down the hall, to the top of the stairs he yelled, "Ok you guys…

you woke her up… and she's still crying… and wants a cup of coffee!" Before I could roll out of bed he was back under the covers curled up against me. I held him until the coffee and the parade of family entered my room. Soon my king size bed was full… and what a sad sight, we all had swollen eyes.

After apologies and lots of hugs, I left our kids making travel arrangements and I caught the first plane to Chicago to be with my mother and Kim's family.

During the flight I tried to plan the day, what do I say to Mom, the kids, how do I keep from crying? Slow deep breaths, slow deep breaths…What would Kim want? How can I make this better? They just witnessed their mother die in front of their young eyes, how do we heal that, and will we ever? I can't cry in front of her kids, I need to comfort them; be strong, no tears… slow deep breaths.

When I arrived my mother made it easy for me. As I reached to embrace her she responded in an angry voice, "I expected you earlier." As I kissed her forehead, I apologized and said, "Mom please I'm doing the best I can." We had an unspoken agreement. She didn't mention too often how I broke her heart when I moved away with her grandchildren, as long as I was there whenever she needed me.

Mom sat stoic in her shade drawn, dark living room. Her petite body held up straight by her wing style chair. On occasion, a single tear would flow down her cheek and disappear into her neckline. She didn't seem to feel it, as she never wiped or brushed it away. "Oh my

God," I thought, "Why is her burden so heavy?" In a seven year timeframe we/Mom lost my Dad to cancer. Her granddaughter died tragically in a car accident. Her mother died a slow death to Alzheimer's. Now her youngest child, a daughter, dies suddenly. When she lost Kim, she lost her best buddy. Life had been especially cruel, her granddaughter, and now her daughter, in a displaced order and sudden tragic deaths.

No family should be as good at making funeral arrangements as we were, unless you're a funeral director. My three young adult sons had assumed the role of pallbearers too many times. More than most will face in a lifetime.

Another difficult part for us was the eulogy. Who would present it? We all felt like a truck hit us. My brother and sisters didn't feel they could do it, nor did I. I did some public speaking when I had to for work; small groups or presentations. However, not without huge amounts of anxiety and under easier circumstance then this.

My husband, an awesome, experienced public speaker was usually our go-to-guy for the eulogies. My heart was nagging me (or maybe Kim's voice in my head) that it should be one of her siblings. That's what she would want, a more personal touch to provide comfort for the kids. Anything we could do to lessen the trauma of this experience needed to be done.

I prayed for strength, and prepared my husband to deliver the eulogy. I even gave his name to our priest. A few minutes before he was to start, I glanced at her three children, ages eleven, nine and seven and their innocent, lost expressions. And I got so mad. "This is just wrong!" I thought, "Our poor kid's my God! My God! They shouldn't be going through this." That anger fueled me with enough adrenalin to deliver her eulogy. When I whispered my plan in my husband's ear, he handed me the notes with an approving smile.

As I stood on the altar, elevated above her flower and satin draped casket, to a church filled to capacity, I took that slow deep breath. Then I smiled and winked at my niece and nephews in the front row. My fears and anger vanished as they smiled back. I told the story of our last phone conversation Kim and I had just a few days before. I recalled how the discussion took an odd turn and we were actually talking about… "This church," I said, "Saint Hubert's, this was our church when we were children too. We made our First Holy Communions here, we were married here, and we baptized our babies here. But in the old days (what kid doesn't like an olden day's story) before this beautiful building was built we held church in the old building next to the church that's now used as the gym. As little girls the summers were so hot, and no one had air conditioning. And together (I drew another breath)… we had the best laugh as we remembered fainting from the heat while in church… cur-plunk… and down we went…as our Sunday dresses went up." There was a short but appropriate amount of laughter. And as I watched her kids giggle in that front row, I knew her spirit was in charge. I was just the vessel, her go-to-guy so to speak. Who knew a conversation about nothing would become so important… and would complete "our" lifetime of laughter together. It had only been a couple of days. Her laughter was still fresh in my heart, soul and mind. I could hear her as I recounted our conversation…

And then before God I opened my broken, but grateful heart, and reminded those that loved her how fortunate we were that she graced our lives for forty-one years. I followed with the promise that her life and memory would live on through her children.

Even today when I'm sad the scent of lilies fills the air around me, her favorite flower. I can feel her bouncing on my lap. She was always more affectionate than me and was blessed with a playful spirit. I was old, before I was old.

The last time I saw her, my Mom threw a party to celebrate my brother's twenty-fifth wedding anniversary. Kim sat next to me at our table as we had dinner. There were lots of laughs sitting with my sisters, but the thing I remember most is how she reached for my hand that night and just held it. If she wasn't holding my hand she was touching my jewelry, my necklace, my earrings, to my watch and then back to holding my hand. I flashed back to when we were kids and she loved to annoy me that way. She would jump on my lap and plant a big kiss on my cheek. That night however I wasn't annoyed, she, for whatever reason, needed to touch me. Who knew it would be the last physical contact between us. As I recall it was slightly awkward, maybe it needed to be, to instill this cherished memory for me.

After the services I had a chance to talk to my uncle. He was a highly respected physician and surgeon. He carefully questioned me about the details we had to that point. I shared the preliminary autopsy report that would be the cause of death on her death certificate. The complete autopsy results wouldn't be available for weeks. "Kim had coronary artery disease and died from a heart attack." I said. His response was, "there is some other anomaly here. A young woman's heart is generally protected by her estrogen levels." He knew our family health history, our grandmother and mother had no history of heart disease. Our dad's family had the cancer history but not heart disease. My uncle, a very distinguished looking man, gently shook his head, adjusted his glasses and looked me directly in the eyes and said, "No Pam, there's some anomaly here."

A couple of weeks later I pulled out my dictionary. I wanted to be sure I understood this rarely used word.

The definition of Anomaly: irregularity, incongruity, difference, variance, glitch, abnormality, inconsistency.

If Kim's life was affected by an anomaly I thought my chances of having the same anomaly were rare. As a result, during the year before my heart attack, any symptom, or warning sign I felt, I attributed to sympathy pains for my sister. She had the anomaly.

Notes from my heart:

What I know for sure, ten years later: When we were kids we rarely had professional medical care. Just about every childhood disease was managed with baby aspirin, or some kind of a salve. We received our immunizations from the health department or stood in line after church for the Polio vaccine. As adult women our response to illness was to take two aspirins and rest, it had served us well for most of our life, until it didn't.

1. Women too often ignore fatigue. Depending how you were raised you might think it's your lot in life, your female responsibility. It's not.

2. We need to become better care givers and listeners for ourselves, our sisters, daughters, mothers and our friends.

3. Women need to create an advocacy support system encouraging one another and expecting the best of medical care for themselves. We insist on it for our children, spouses, and parents.

4. A constant mild fatigue alone is enough to warrant a check-up.

5. Learning to be more protective of yourself and your energy is difficult, but critical.

6. Whether it's your own personal health crisis or the loss of a loved one, laughter is still one of the best medicines. Give yourself permission laugh again and find reasons to. Watch a

funny sitcom, buy a joke book. "Laughter Therapy" massages internal organs and stimulates hormones that release endorphins known to provide a sense of relaxation and well-being.

7. Depending what you read, there are still many doctors that believe female hearts are protected by their estrogen levels. Maybe that's true for some. Both my sister and I were still having regular menstrual cycles when we had our heart attacks.

8. You could never cry enough or hurt enough to change life's realities; a heart attack or a death. It's done.

9. If you're so inclined prayer is a powerful weapon against sadness.

10. For most mothers, all aspects of family life seem to flow through us. With today's life styles it's hundreds of details. It's okay to say no sometimes and simply slow down the family activity. You don't have to be on every committee and the kids don't need to play every seasonal sport.

Chapter 3:
A Case of Denial

"There are no mistakes, no coincidences. All events are blessings given to us to learn from." —*Dr. Wayne Dyer*

The night of my heart attack the Cardiologist on duty (that injected my clot buster) questioned me about earlier symptoms; "Did you have any chest pain or tightness prior to this night," "Yes" I said, "Tightness, I thought my bras were too tight." "Did you experience shortness of breath?" He asked, and again I responded, "Yes, I thought I was experiencing mild panic attacks because my sister died." "Oh I'm so sorry" he responded, "When and how did she die." He asked. "Just about two years ago, she had a fatal heart attack; she was only forty one years old." I responded. "She was so young, I'm sorry," he continued, "Have you experienced unusual fatigue?" He asked. Again I responded, "Yes, I felt like the earth was trying to draw me in, but I've been so busy you see, working full time, going back and forth to Chicago trying to help with my sisters family." "Have you had any other problems?" He asked, again I responded, "Yes, I've had a lot of low back pain and leg pains." "When was the last time you saw your doctor?" "A year ago or so, I had an episode of bronchitis." Did you report these problems to your doctor? "No" I responded, "I took two aspirin and usually felt better."

You would think the loss of my sister would have spurred my interest into a preventive or proactive state of mind. I should have been researching the possible implications to my life or for a better understanding of her death. But I didn't. I was so heartbroken losing her and drowning in an emotional crisis. There wasn't time to address anything else but what formed in my path. And there was plenty to do. As a result, I remained truly ignorant to the female warning signs. I expected that something so serious would come with great pain. I had greater pains in child birth, monthly cycles, tooth aches, etc. This heart attack was confusing; it was gentle aches and pain that radiated my body. None of the symptoms prevented me from talking, laughing, eating, driving or walking. I just didn't feel good and then, I died.

I couldn't handle one more thing and never imagined the power of this emotion, denial. Before I experienced it up close and personal, it was just a word, used in association with others. Although, it found a home in my vocabulary and was tied to so many feelings I couldn't accept. If I had shared this anomaly with my sister, was my only fate an early death as well? If I survived the anomaly, why would "I" be given special grace when she didn't? I had already developed a survivor's guilt without the anomaly in the mix. It was just easier to reject the whole idea.

When I heard the gentle voices in my head that whispered, "You need to go to the doctor," I responded with, "You're a hypochondriac; all your aches and pains are ridiculous." When the voice got louder, so did I. "What are you going to tell him, it hurts sometimes here and sometimes over here? He'll send you to the psych ward." It worked until I was brought to my knees in surrender.

I used the anomaly to hide behind. I felt a sense of safety there. At some level, it was probably a healthy coping mechanism. It allowed me more time to deal with the grief. When someone says you're in denial, it usually means you aren't being honest with yourself or about something in your life. The truth and life's realities were more than I was able to mentally absorb. Thoughts were rejected more often than selected. Although it may appear obvious to those around you, while you're in denial, I was not consciously aware of my behavior. It is much easier to understand ten years later.

A definite negative is when it prevents you from effectively dealing with issues that need attention. Not uncommon, it's a reaction to trauma. By denying the existence of a problem we dispel the need to cope with it until life forces the issue.

You don't usually or consciously decide to be in denial, it is often an unconscious event as the research suggests.

After the angioplasty and a placement of a stent I was told by the Cardiologist that released me from the hospital I'd probably live to be eighty five and I'd be as good as new after a month or so of rest. "Normally" he said, "the recovery time from an angioplasty and stent is only a few days, but the recovery time from the heart attack is significantly longer. See how you feel. Discuss it with your personal Cardiologist; you can most likely return to work in four to six weeks." He handed me the American Heart Association's guide for any further questions I might have. I was warned against heavy lifting, if I remember correctly nothing over five pounds. That ruled out picking up the grandchildren for a while. Then he told me I should never shovel snow again. "Oh darn it," I replied. "How about pumping gasoline-I hate that even more?" He laughed.

Notes from my heart:

What I know for sure ten years later: My life was spared by my sister's death. I believe my sister was completely blindsided by her symptoms, she had no form of reference. She was a busy mom that had been tired, developed a stomach ache making dinner, went to her bedroom to lie down for a few minutes and died. My son had the benefit of this knowledge and the unforgettable heart ache of carrying the casket of his beloved aunt. He also had the presence of mind when he found out I was sick to say "what if?"

1. How many pain relievers do you take in a day or a week? Don't ignore your aches and pains they are symptoms. My leg and back pain were probably due to poor circulation, it disappeared when they stented my coronary artery.

2. If your bra feels too tight and you haven't had any weight gain, that tightness probably has a different cause.

3. We often justify our aches and pains with our busy schedules, however if our lives are causing us physical discomfort that alone is cause for concern, investigation and adjustment.

4. Frequent or severe shortness of breath should never be ignored

5. How do you separate denial from reality? I'm not sure you can always accomplish this on your own. Pose the question to a trusted relative or friend and honestly examine their re-

sponse. You might be very surprised at what other eyes may see.

6. When you're ready, try to return to an abbreviated schedule of your life. But enter it with a trial and error attitude, if it's too difficult; try again in a week or two. Remember to pace yourself, the race is over. The goal is recovery and survival.

7. I should have protected my heart better, when a feeling of sadness is your most dominant emotion; that constant drain will surely lead to physical illness.

8. How long is too long to be in mourning is individual. Most experts say a year. From my own experience, I believe sudden deaths are a traumatic event and should be addressed differently. Most churches and many cities offer grief support groups.

9. I suggested counseling for everyone but myself. I should have asked for help. There's no shame in seeking counseling.

Chapter 4:
At the Banks of Grace

"Believers, look up-take courage. The Angels are nearer than you think." —Dalai Lama

I guess you could literally say I was a heart attack waiting to happen. That fatal level of denial surely would have led to my demise as I slept that night, if not for God. One of my core beliefs is; if you live your life giving more than you take, in your day of need you can draw from a "Grace" account. My "Grace" withdrawal was complete with all the bells and whistles of a creative drama; swallowing those aspirins and keeping my blood just thin enough to move it through that barely opened artery. My "Knight in Shining Armor," (my Brian) miraculously appears in time to take me to the safe arms in the emergency room. My favorite part was the choice of settings; to have a heart attack and die surrounded by medical staff, duly equipped with a crash cart. Now that's a perfectly orchestrated plan, complete with a happy ending. ...*Thank you God.*

Who was this person I had become? At what point did I lose the healthy mind/ body connection that I had cultivated throughout my life? You may have heard someone say; before their illness they felt their life spin out of control. This is not a cliché, it's very real. I was in constant motion, without focus, I moved from one problem to another, my thoughts were scrambled. This is the state of mind that permitted the denial and the illness in.

Warning Sign: When laughter hurts, you're in trouble.

If something moved me to the point of laughter you could bet it would also produce tears. The harder I laughed the more I choked back the tears. Kim's death alone was enough to cause havoc in my life, and it had been closely preceded by the loss of three other loved ones. Although on the surface, I appeared to be the solid, stable person that many depended on. Inside I was suffering, and had at least a low grade depression. Though quite functional, and with a vacant smile, I tried desperately to care for the needs of my family. At that time three of our kids were teenagers, with all the problems common and associated to their growth. Work, home, our aging parents, the support role of grandparenthood, and helping my sister's family whenever possible, created such an imbalance. Juggling life was hard enough, but now I was dodging death.

When I told the Interventional Cardiologist, "Death is not an option for me," (like I was purchasing a new car or something) I was really pleading for my life, but not born out of a personal fear of death. I really wanted to grab him by the white coat and say, "Look Doc our family has been through enough pain and suffering! My mother can't lose another child! Do you understand me? Do you? Do you? You must find some way to keep me alive!"

My world held an abundance of strong loving bonds to my husband, children, and grandchildren. I'm so blessed. Our love and the power of their energy kept a strong grip on me, they called me home. Do not underestimate the power of visualization combined with determination. First I prayed for my life. The rest of that car ride to the hospital, I visualized myself at my grandson's baptisms and willed myself into the audience as my daughter received her diploma. And that memory of despair in her eyes… that sole tear flowing down her check…I was sustained by my devotion to her, my first love, my Mom. Nothing else was going to hurt her, not if I could help it.

I never missed a week calling my Mom. Every weekend we'd spend at least an hour catching up on the week's news. She'd always begin our conversation with, "So what's going on in the Land of Oz." And my kids always provided plenty of material for us to laugh about. She would patiently await my call but, rarely called me. When the kids asked if they should call her after my heart attack I said, "Absolutely not. I will call her this weekend as planned, under no circumstances." I warned, "Do you call her."

Well she must have had a moment of 'mother's intuition,' and out of the clear blue sky called my home. Of course she wanted to speak to me. Our youngest daughter tripped all over herself and then confessed, "Grandma, Moms in the hospital." After a long pause her response was, "Ask your mother to call me," and then she quickly said, "Goodbye." No how's she doing? What's wrong with her?

When I returned her call, and started to explain she hung up on me. I waited a minute called her back and she let it ring forever, finally she answered, "Mom," I said, "We need to talk about this." "No we don't, I need to put my groceries away," she said. "Goodbye Pamela."

"Mom… Mom… please Mom do not hang up again," I pleaded, "Mom I had a little procedure I'm going to be fine." She responded with "Good! Then call me this weekend I'm busy." "Okay Mom I will." We never discussed it again.

My Mom's denial was so strong it allowed her to completely reject the reality of my heart attack- after watching her youngest daughter stripped from her arms by the same disease. Her mind couldn't absorb another shock. Her denial allowed her to have some sense of control of her already vulnerable existence. While at times I was frightened, and wished I could talk to her about it, I found peace in knowing she was protected from yet another hurt.

Notes from my heart:

The wish list: *These following heart notes are what I know now and what I wish I would have done then, that might have prevented the heart attack.*

1. Had a complete medical check up

2. Sought the help and counsel of a nutritionist

3. Started vitamin therapy

4. Received private grief counseling

5. Talked to my priest or spiritual counselor

6. Took a yoga or tai chi class for stress reduction and spiritual connection.

7. Started a walking program.

8. Did something to pamper myself at least one hour a week. Get a massage or visit an old beautiful cathedral for solitude and prayer.

9. Explored meditation and breathing practices

10. I wish I knew about guided imaginary

11. Turned the music back on, for some reason I stopped doing the things I enjoyed. I couldn't concentrate well enough to

read or even watch television, but music might have been able to penetrate the mental confusion.

12. I wish I would have reprioritized, rather than trying to be everywhere for everyone. I wish I had hired some help to get me through the surge of needs.

When you examine this list you'll realize just giving myself/yourself an hour each day and an additional hour "special time" once a week would have made a huge difference in the quality of life. It may not have prevented the heart disease, but possibly may have prevented a heart attack.

Chapter 5:
There's No Place Like Home

"Change your thoughts and you change your world."
—Reverend Billy Graham

When you're engaged in a life crisis as I was, one might think that normal daily life problems would cease to exist, at least temporarily. They don't. Just days after my heart attack, while recovering at home, our home was hit by lightening. A satellite dish was not grounded properly (four years before) when it was mounted. It suddenly, became a lightning rod. The lightening hit the house with such force it cracked the underground water main. To repair it, they needed heavy equipment to dig up my beautifully landscaped front yard to reach the pipe. Why now? What a sight.

When they restored our water the upstairs toilet overflowed in our kid's bathroom. No one thought to turn off the toilets water source. Their remedy was to take my best bath towels and cover the floor. No one told me, until later when the water started to seep through the ceiling into the family room of my model perfect home. As the ceiling collapsed I thought about how I would entertain in five days. That was the weekend; two of my grandsons were to be baptized, with a party to follow at our home.

It was probably a good thing that I was over medicated. I would have been a wreck trying to plan our family celebrations. It was the end of May and our schedules were full with family events. A week later we were expecting house guests (my mom and sister) for our daughters high school graduation. No pressure. We had planned yet another celebration afterwards at our home. Luckily, I've always enjoyed entertaining. It became a necessity with the size of our family and young ages of our grandchildren. No one wanted to go to a restaurant with all the babies.

My husband was very supportive. Every night after dinner he'd walk with me. Or keep me company while I was on the treadmill. He was always encouraging me to do more of an incline or go faster. "Yeah, you really think that's the answer for me," I'd ask? He was trying to train me for a marathon-I was trying to survive. I was so weak.

While he sat drinking a beer, I ask myself what's wrong with this picture. He's the one with high blood pressure; I never had high blood pressure. All those years that he ate junk food at night, I'd grab a piece of fruit. He ate steak; I'd have soup and salad. He was definitely the Type "A" personality, I was his opposite. I stopped to smell the roses he stopped only to buy them. He was always in a hurry; I'd remind him it's Sunday why do we need to rush today?

He did however have a remarkable ability to shut down and block out his surroundings. How does he do it? I recall watching him relaxing in his favorite overstuffed chair. He was seemingly oblivious to the huge hole in the ceiling above him. *When I grow up I want to be more like him I thought*. Here you see our absolute opposite personalities. In matters of the house/home and family, I'm let's just say… more engaged. Yeah, that's a nice way to put it…more engaged.

Those lightning strike sayings danced around in my head. You know; "may I be struck down by lightning if"…Well, they held a new meaning when my home was hit by lightening. Especially following three jolts of electricity to my restart my heart only a week before. And I tried not to take the family room ceiling caving in as a sign, or a personal attack either. But, I need to tell you it was difficult. I had lived long enough to experience plenty of storms in my life, you get through them. However in the past I entered the storm physically and mentally stronger. This test seemed unfair. Chaos seemed to be swirling around me. Nothing made sense. There was to be no peace or rest for me.

Likewise, my kids were engaged in testing me as well. I mentioned we have five kids. The three that were still home I lovingly nicknamed, My Brainy Bunch. When they were tested in school they all achieved test scores in the top percentiles in the country. Along with their Dad they all enjoyed IQ's in the superior range, only a point or two different between them. While they'd all kicked butt in the game of Jeopardy, general life management was a challenge for this group. If you want to feel dumb watch Jeopardy with them, collectively they knew all the answers. If you wanted to feel like a genius live with them.

My oldest daughter tried to explain her dilemma to me; why her Bachelors Degree may take five years rather than four. "Let me remove that barrier from your thought process." I recommended. "Find a way to accomplish it in four years or find a way to pay for the fifth year. The cost is running about $12,000.00 per year. Honey, it's your choice."

Our son received notice of academic probation and when I inquired, "WHY?" He stated, "His classes didn't hold his interest." I found out later he majored in shooting pool that semester. When he wasn't in the on-campus pool hall, he rented movies from two different video stores. The stores would call the house constantly for the movies to be returned and the threat of astronomical late fees. Oh, the best part was when he returned all the movies to the wrong stores. It was constant confusion.

More than a threat to my intelligence was when the car that we bought him blew up; because he neglected to put oil in it. I have a saying that I often impart to my children and grandchildren: "My money is a terrible thing to waste." He was given an ultimatum. "You have one week to find a full-time job, and I recommend that you find it on a bus line that can transport you to and from work." Then I presented him with a bill for that wasted semester. When he complained, I stooped to a deviation of that rather effective line our parents often used. "Keep it up; I'll add the cost of the car to that bill."

It had become a family tradition with the Brainy Bunch to graduate from high school early. That same week, our youngest child, kept with tradition and was graduating at sixteen, following in the footsteps of her brother and sister. She felt the need to let me know that none of her friends were virgins. She decided she shouldn't be either. It was her time. "Please Mom don't try to stop me. You raised a really good kid. Look how long I waited, for you."

"For me…! Jesus, Mary and Joseph… Child…this isn't about me?" I continued. "I also raised a beautiful, intelligent person who surely must realize that you don't need to achieve all your milestones in the same week! You know it's not a prerequisite to have sex before college!" With certain kids loud is better. "Oh Mom," she said, "And please don't tell Daddy that I'm thinking about this, because men are really funny about these things."

My oldest son came to check up on me and found me taking a nap. He said, "So this is your new look, junky clothes, no makeup and you think you can get away with this, why… because you died?" Our family comedian had me laughing most of the afternoon. Another smart guy, he coaxed me out of bed to the stove to feed his body, while he nourished my soul with laughter.

And then there's Brian, my kid with the best timing. He's the only one that understood that the family room ceiling was causing me great anxiety. Let alone the mountain of dirt on the front lawn. He would call every morning to make sure I was alive. After work he came over and made the repairs. Plus he made sure he wasn't working alone, he took charge of that house with a drill sergeant quality. And he kept his brother and sisters working alongside of him.

Unfortunately, someone else was able to pick up on the anxiety levels in that house. Our granddaughter, only two years old, but born with an old soul. Our precious gift that came into the world just two months after my sister Kim died. Shortly after my heart attack, she started to stutter. Until that moment she was a happy healthy child, and a very early talker. We sought help for her immediately. We found her vocabulary was so advanced for her age, that her mouth was having trouble keeping up with her brain. She needed more Barney songs, and less conversation with all the superior IQ's. Amen, me too...

So what do you do? When the loves of your life, your family, become energy drains? Especially under those circumstances when my sole focus should have been rest and recovery. Yet, I was surrounded by love, devotion and total chaos. What-do you-do?

During her visit my sister suggested that I go to a good health spa for a couple of weeks. I guess she felt the energy too. "I can't leave my family!" I protested. By profession she is a registered nurse and of course put my health under the microscope. After a short study of the interaction between me and my husband she said, "You two are complete opposites and, you do realize he causes you stress?" "Yes," I replied, "But only if I let him. And you know, a few of our kids are very much like him, and I can't send them back either."

She worked for a large well known teaching hospital in Chicago. She would discuss my case with their Head of Cardiology; he was always in agreement with the medications and the procedures I was receiving. There were times during this process that a second opinion was a great comfort.

To find me taking a nap in the middle of the afternoon as my son did, was a rarity. The event must have frightened him. I felt pretty beaten that week. I remember the conversation I had with myself and God…

"I'm tired of being a Mom; I don't want to do it anymore. I'm out numbered. Their Dad travels too much. I tired of doing it alone. I feel like a single parent most of the time. Maybe I shouldn't take their behavior so personally. They are older now. I could pretend were all roommates. Yeah, that's it; I'll view them as roommates, and involve myself only when I want to, kind of like a hobby. I really enjoy being a grandmother though. Maybe I'll just do that. Look, even that's on a fast track; four grandchildren in five years. We're already having double baptisms. My husband is always in a hurry, he always rushing me. Lord I can't seem to move fast enough or think fast enough. Am I having a mental break down too? Summers here, I can't travel to Chicago right now; I'll need to bring Kim's kids to me. Oh no, how am I going to keep this heart attack a secret from them. That's all they need. They're going to want to do the summertime stuff, amusement parks. Great, can you imagine yourself on a roller coaster right now? Heck woman you're already on one. And I'll be cleared to return to work in a month or so, terrific. I'm sure I let out a sigh as I fell asleep."

Sometimes you need to put your feelings into words so you can hear just how stupid it all sounds. I loved my life and I loved my family. When my son woke me out of my temporary escape I remembered how deeply I loved them. They were my joy, and my purpose. He was my first born and I saw the desperation in his eyes through all the jokes. His actions were, come on Mom, hang on, I'm here, and we're going to get you through this. In hind sight the behavior of all five our kids was an attempt to draw me closer to them. Whether to say Mom I need you. Please keep our train on the tracks. We need your advice to move forward. My older sons had the benefit of our years together and wanted nothing more than to protect me. We all held on to each other, for more time.

Although I mention more than once how I enjoyed this cosmetically lovely home, and it was. It was so much more than beautiful surroundings. It was also a safe haven for our family, it's where our kids were all adored and made to feel special. A home to be sure that they were all proud of, as they always filled it with their friends. They were encouraged to speak their mind and share their problems. I got what I asked for. These were prayers answered, not punishments. When the lightning cracked the water main it didn't affect the foundation we built our home on. And I don't mean the concrete base. There was no damage to the spiritual foundation of our home life and family. The very core was built on love, faith and respect. Prayer was and is my weapon of choice.-Through prayer I was reminded that there wasn't a problem too great that couldn't be resolved by this family. I just needed to ask. Those meals I was concerned about, my oldest son was a Chef by trade; he made awesome meals for us. There was no one more detail oriented than Brian managing the house and repairs. My Brainy Bunch took care of the fine points of party planning; it was good for me to let go and let someone else pick the flowers, arrange the tables, prepare the house for company, and do the shopping.

The kids meet the standards I set, and were prepared for my Mom's arrival. I felt very grateful and proud of them. They did hear me more often than I thought. But was I prepared? Remember I wasn't sick. And she made sure to treat me as such too. Shortly after her arrival she told me I could use a good hair cut, needed to lose some weight and asked, "Have you been to the dentist lately Honey?" Kim had a nickname/saying for Mom; she called her, "Crazy Shirl, that's my girl." As I was being tortured by her not so constructive criticism, in my mind I wandered off and shared a laugh with Kim, "Yep… that's our girl." And then I responded to my mother by telling her how lovely she looked.

Now years later, I'm able to view that time with a higher degree of wisdom and humor. While I enjoy cooking it's okay to let someone else do it on occasion. I needed to learn, not every aspect, nor every ache, pain or heartache that these kids experience was somehow my fault or responsibility. I think I was on high alert for so long because the Brainy Bunch seemed to make unwise choices in spite of our efforts. My maternal instinct wanted to protect them. When it came to home and family I had developed that type "A" personality. There's no way I could have died that week. Who would have told the kids what to wear to my funeral? We had exposed the kids to as much as we could. Sometimes life is the best teacher. I needed to trust my efforts. Pray, and let it be.

Notes from my heart:

What I know for sure, ten years later: Sometimes divine direction comes from people that inspire you, or simply aggravate you; those that force you to think or push you to a new level of awareness. Everyone in my life had a purpose or reminded me of my purpose.

1. Learning to let go of some responsibilities, even temporarily should be a priority. When you're feeling better you can always resume where you left off.

2. A health spa might be a great idea for some.

3. I'm one of those people that need to get slapped upside the head, before I stop and assess the situation. I needed to be placed in total chaos before I made sensible changes. If there was ever a time to rethink your life course it's now.

4. Ask your family for help, they want to support you.

5. To avoid stresses between you and family members try to be very specific as to what you need or expect.

6. Don't assume they know how to do something you never let them do before.

7. Remember their frightened too.

8. Allow time for family discussions about the illness.

9. Encourage them to walk with you. I've had some of my best discussions taking a walk.

10. Watch out for the energy drains, have a plan to cope with them or not.

11. I was so sure that I didn't have any type "A" personality tendencies until I really took a serious look at my behavior. Maybe you call it perfectionism, is it? Or does it border on obsession. I don't know too many obsessions that are without stressful feelings or emotions. I preferred to refer to mine as a passion but when I became obsessed with each minuscule detail, it was exhausting. That's not passion.

12. Insist on peace in your home.

13. Personally, I do not believe you get sick from being too busy. If you're doing the things you love everyday and you're happy and full of passion, but that's not usually how life works. It's all the dreaded responsibilities and the constant stress of having to manage it all. You must reprioritize and rethink all daily activities to find balance and a less stressful environment.

Chapter 6:
Be Still and Know God

"Health is the greatest gift, contentment the greatest wealth, faithfulness the best relationship." —*Mother Teresa*

We survived the repairs, baptisms, graduation, house guest and our celebrations. Just as we started to see the new growth of grass where the dirt pile was, I felt the tingling in my left arm return. It radiated through my shoulder down my left arm. Before I could regain my energy, I had a reaction to the stent. It was only three weeks after the heart attack. The process is called restenosis whereby scar tissue forms around the stent and closes the artery. Between the scar tissue and all these new medications that were prescribed for me I was tired, cold and numb most of the time. I could barely finish a sentence, let alone a thought.

To this day, I remember questioning the amount of medication prescribed for me after my heart attack. I don't even know how I eventually went back to work, made a decision or drove my car. I'm sure I was still traumatized from my death experience. The medication certainly didn't provide clarity. My Cardiologist insisted these were, "The gold standard, the proven drugs after a heart attack." Thankfully, he also listened when I told him I could not function from the medication. He then very slowly and carefully cut back on my prescribed dose to a more manageable dose. However, he insisted I stay on them for my own protection and I heeded his advice. By nature I question everything; I'm just not easily compliant. In this case I often found myself opposing the prescribed medical interventions. As medicated as I was, I could still hear my gut. And my gut said, "This was not the right course of treatment for me." The situation was more than difficult; being so dependent on this doctor's wisdom to get me through the complications. In my defense after a month I was supposed to be feeling better. Well on my road to recovery. But I wasn't. Was it due to the closing artery? Was I over medicated?

In his defense, ten years ago, the care protocol was certainly strongly based on male history. I say that without criticism. It's a fact, and I just didn't respond well to that current standard of care. I believe that Cardiology Team was at the forefront in technology for heart care at that point in time.

Before I went back to the Cardiac Catherization Lab, they ran some tests. I wore a Holter Monitor, (tests the heart for beat irregularities) for a few days, then I was scheduled for a stress test, an echocardiogram, and the results were fine.

The day of my heart attack my first symptom was a feeling of doom, overwhelming and distinct. Thankfully, with each complication I experienced that year it was always accompanied by that feeling. It became my warning signal, a heart detector. The ache in my left arm and tingling sensation in both arms started first. However within days the doom would take over. It's a difficult feeling to describe; I literally felt my light going out.

My fate would surely have taken a different course for my family, had my Cardiologist not responded to me when I said "Doc something's wrong." Or worse, "Doc something's wrong again." And in spite of the good test results, thank God he listened to me.

And throughout my storm just as my light would dim a life boat would appear and row me to safety.

Just weeks after my heart attack I was back in the Cardiac Catherization Lab for placement of another stent (#2) and clearing of scar tissue. As before I was awake during the beginning of the procedure and was able to see on the screen the closure of the artery as they put the dye in. It's amazing that something so tiny causes such a problem and is the passage to life or death. At some point during the procedure he would ask if I was comfortable. Although, it didn't seem to matter what my response was. I can remember saying I feel an ache or that I was fine and either way at that point, he put me to sleep. My guess is that's when the stent went in. Shortly after that, I'd wake up in recovery.

Somewhere after stent #2 my entire family became more aware of their own behavior and mindful of the moment. Just as I questioned what I might have done to cause the second stent-they looked inside of themselves with the same question. When I survived the heart attack they accepted the miracle and ran with it. It was as though they preferred to close that chapter quickly. It was over, they had their Mom back. But when my life was threatened with the second stent, life changed for all of us. Suddenly I was viewed and treated as fragile. They were more careful and supportive and some of them had their first arguments with God.

However even in a more peaceful place, my body was reacting quickly to the stents. Two months later the same scenario, I had another angioplasty of the scar tissue and placement of another stent (#3). Thank God my Cardiologist was still listening. He didn't send me for the tests again, instead scheduled me promptly into the Cardiac Catherization Lab.

He'd always asked if I was feeling depressed. My response was always the same, "I have good days and great days. I'd ask if it was time for me to start cardiac rehab; he'd ask about my daily exercise. I was walking out doors (at a leisurely pace) about two miles daily and/or on the tread mill. I'd ask what my heart rate goal should be; he'd say don't pay any attention to that for now, your heart rate is being controlled by the medication. He'd ask what I was eating; I'd say "oatmeal and salmon." He'd laugh. And during the car ride home, I'd cry.

I asked my family doctor why he thought my Cardiologist hadn't prescribed the cardiac rehab yet. His response was, "I don't think you're well enough, and I concur with him, you've had serious complications." No one tried to keep information from me, I'm not sure I always understood what questions I should ask. However, my doctors never spoke about the restenosis with confidence.

At one point, I remember hearing the concern in my Cardiologists voice and witnessed the sorrow in his eyes when he said, "Pam I can't seem to heal you." At that moment I thought, "Heal me?" I never expected him to heal me. Healing was an act of *Grace* that would be spontaneous; a gift from God I thought, through my body, mind, and soul. His purpose was to keep me alive and he accomplished that to the best of his ability.

Months into maneuvering the storm, I was still seeking divine intervention. And my prayers for guidance constantly flooded my thoughts. By the Grace of God, as we were running out of options the FDA approved a clinical trial. I was one of the first people in Maryland approved for the trial, in January 2001. The procedure was called Brachytherapy; they placed a bead of radiation in my coronary artery and that was to prevent further restenosis. With three more stents: numbers 4, 5, & 6, almost eight months after my heart attack, I was grateful to be alive.

I was unhappy that my Cardiologist could not perform the procedure; I felt safe with him. However, only the doctors involved in that clinical trial had the training, therefore the authority. I was surprised to wake from the procedure to the news that I received three more stents. I later questioned my Cardiologist and was told that the decision was made to treat women more aggressively.

This became my never ending night mare. In my stillness between procedures, during the procedures, and attempts of recovering from them, I worshipped. I needed divine energy to sustain my hope and faith. When you're "in spirit," conversation and attitudes are lifted to a higher realm. Rather than why me, I heard why not me. Health problems can occur at any age. Hold your head up high this crisis won't last. Staying in faith prevented the onset of bitterness.

After each procedure I had to lie still for hours with a weight on my leg to prevent movement. My monitors would sound constantly, due a drop in my blood pressure. It would remain alarmingly low until I was allowed to get up and move around. Usually the nurses would come in, appearing more annoyed each time, make an adjustment, they'd ask how I was doing and then leave.

This time however I think they sent an Angel disguised as a nurse. She appeared to have all the answers for what I had been praying for. She came in response to my monitor alarm, and while she was resetting it, she proceeded to ask a series of questions. Why was I there, who was my Cardiologist, what medications was I on, did I take any vitamin supplements...On the record she said my Cardiologist was one of the best in the area. The other best was the doctor that just performed my Brachytherapy, "so you have the two best Interventional Cardiologists in the state, you're lucky, that's good." She said.

Off the record she suggested that there is Alternative Care available. This was not part of your Cardiologists medical training and as a result they aren't able to provide it. They are tending only to your heart, "Who's addressing your overall health." She asked. I thought for a minute about my family doctor, but unless I had an infection he was useless, while I was under the care of the Cardiologist. These multiply stents and procedures were not common, and I became a bit of an enigma. He referred my every ache and pain back to the Cardiologist, so indeed she was correct. Who was tending to my overall health?

She recommended that I see a Nutritionist and gave me a website of a doctor (Dr. Sinatra on the "QT", she advised, this is against hospital protocol) he specializes in female heart issues. She saw on the table the heart booklet the hospital had provided. She handed me the book and a pen to take some notes. "Write this down"…then she quickly thumbed through it. When she got to the back page she showed me the flyer insert on their newly formed Complementary Care Clinic. "Yes this is good, after you get home call them, they are doing some really important work there. They can refer you to a Nutritionist too," she said. Then she said, "This isn't my floor I need to get back to my patients," and in a flash she was gone.

Upon my release from the hospital I went home and followed her instructions. My first call was to the Complementary Care Clinic. It was their protocol that the first appointment was with the Director. After his assessment I would be directed to the necessary care providers. Unfortunately, I had to wait two weeks to meet with him.

Notes from my heart:

What I know for sure, ten years later. I refused to allow myself time to be sick. I did everything in my power to resume my normal activities; to send a message and relieve the fears of my family. I needed to give myself permission to be sick so, I could get well. I kept trying to get to third base without moving through second base.

1. It's a common practice today as it was ten years ago to have an angioplasty and stent procedure on a Friday and the following Monday, depending on your line of work be cleared to return to work. For some people this is too soon. I did it, but in retrospect it was too soon for me. We all heal differently, take the time you need.

2. Today they have drug (antibiotic) coated stents; I understand they are having improved results, with less restenosis. If timing allows, discuss with your doctor before you get into the Cardiac Catherization Lab what the plan is.

3. Does your doctor listen to you? Ask how their team or office will manage your emergency calls.

4. Don't be afraid to make a change if you're not getting the care you think you need. At the risk of sounding dramatic it really can be a matter of life or death.

5. Research and understand the purpose and side effects of all prescribed medications. Discuss all the side effects you're experiencing with your doctor.

6. Keep a list in your wallet of all medications and prescribed dose. You'll often need it.

7. Make sure to make your doctor aware of any vitamins or supplements you're taking.

8. Depression is common after both heart attacks and strokes. Please seek the help of a medical professional.

9. Whether you choose an MD, DO, or an ND you'll need whole body care, more than most Cardiologist will provide.

10. Your options for Alternative care shouldn't be presented like an underground secret as mine was. Introduce your Cardiologist to the options you're having success with. Maybe they'll pass it on to other patients.

Chapter 7:
I Am

"No one can make you feel inferior without your consent."
—Eleanor Roosevelt

Most family's trees are filled with the stories of our ancestors that migrated here to build a better life. They were *positive* their journey to America would provide opportunity. Here they would create the life they had only dreamed about: *hope*d for. They came with a *vision*. They had *goals*. They believed in something they couldn't see yet: *faith*. No sacrifice too great for the cause, the family: *love*. If we simply study their behavior, their work ethic, they also gave us the blueprint to build successful businesses and significant lives. Many of the terms used here, could describe a good business or marketing plan. More importantly many are the very heart of *"The Bible"* or *"The Torah."* They define the mindset of that generation.

Yet somehow in the mid 1970's, I found myself defending participation in a Positive Attitude Seminar. Some of my friends and relatives described it as voodoo or cult worship. Was this negative thought process a natural progression of the time? It was popular in the 1960's to question everything. Did it evolve into a culture of suspicion by the 70's? In reality the only thing that was new, was the terminology. The behavior was our inheritance, our foundation, as demonstrated by the generations before us. Who's more *positive* than a person that creates something out of nothing?

By the time I was in my early twenties (ouch over thirty years ago) I was divorced, had two sons under the age of three, and worked fulltime to provide for us. When one of the investors of the restaurant company I worked for, offered a two day seminar in positive thinking and meditation practices. He was a successful psychologist and a motivational speaker. Not only was it free, he enticed us with a promise that we would reap financial benefits with a positive attitude. My biggest problem was childcare. When he offered multiple options for the two-day sessions all the single moms got together and worked out babysitting schedules to attend.

I suspect it's in my DNA. I was fascinated by the thought of what was touted the new age of thinking.

While everyone has a story, restaurant staffs are complete with the dysfunctional childhoods, battered woman, addictions, and an air of low self esteem. There's also the higher education element of many idle degrees awaiting those still in search of "self." Whatever our excuse was, most of us could have benefited from private sessions.

For me personally, the two day session changed my life. What little I had been exposed to from my modest Mid-West up bringing; family, the public school system and church, all told me what to think. These sessions taught me how to think. It awakened the tried and true beliefs I had already formed in my own young life process. It also encouraged the development of your inner guidance system.

The group favorite was the mind/body connection, and the importance of self dialogue. Within minutes of introducing these concepts, the group understood the connection and the stories began.

The most memorable for me, was told by a middle age woman, juggling six kids by herself. She told the group how she repeatedly said throughout the day, "I can't stand it." This became her standard line. It was her expression of anger or happiness. When someone shared something humorous with her, she'd respond with laughter and "I can't stand it." When she was angry with the kids for not doing their chores or homework, she used the same response without the laughter. Until the day she woke up and could not stand up due to severe pain in her legs. She had developed blood clots in both legs. Her hospital stay provided her with a much needed rest and time for reflection. She instinctively wondered if she may have, in part, caused her illness. Her stress levels were off the charts. She ate only at work to save money for food the kids. She was sleep deprived and the words that frequented her vocabulary were closely matched to her emotions; "I can't stand it." Her story stimulated similar, genuine and heartfelt stories from the group.

Throughout this session the class became the teachers as we shared our mind/body connection experiences and the teacher (the psychologist) became the facilitator as he guided us to accept our own, "Physician heal thyself" possibility.

Nurturing my own health is usually prompted into action by a life crisis. For months after my niece died in a horrible car accident I felt like I had the flu. There was no antibiotic able to cure what I had, nor was I able to wrap my mind around losing her. There is no greater tragedy than burying our children. And I ran from the hurt. I couldn't stop moving until the day I found myself in the doctor's office with a lump on the back of my neck and a raging fever. He asked me how long I'd been sick and I said, "Months." He of course questioned my reference to, "Months," and I quickly replied, "No these symptoms are new, but I haven't felt well in months." His second question was, "Have you been under any stress?" "I'm not sure you can call this stress, its sadness, my niece died a few months ago." And as I released those words from my mouth the tears welled in my eyes, it was the beginning of my coming to grips with the grief.

The fever forced me to just lie in bed for days. My job was to rest, think, and recover from my swollen lymph glands. My body was hard at work fighting the infections. My mind moved through the pain. There was to be no recovery without doing the work; and walking through the pain was part of that, it gave me permission to live. The infection was a four or five day recovery, but it took years to find peace in my heart and soul. However, I set the healing in motion that week.

The moment my Cardiologist said he couldn't heal me my fighter spirit took over. He reminded me of my role. How many times in my life had I already released myself on myself, with those three words,- "Physician heal thyself." This time however I was in a different league, and my inner physician was intimidated by the illness: the heart. By comparison, any other health issue I conquered to date seemed trivial. Then I asked myself a question, was I ready to die, because living had become so difficult? Instantly a thunderous NO pierced my thoughts. The problem was my body had been compromised and fragile for too long. There were many months prior, during, and post heart attack that the self dialog was: I feel like I'm dying. This message and feeling that started as a slow leak grew into a relentless companion. I truly believe correcting this self-conversation would not have been possible without the final adjustments made to my medication. Until then I didn't have complete control of my thoughts or my mind.

With a reduction in the medication I regained my mental clarity and was able to understand my role in recovery. For the most part, under the influence of medication, I moved blindly through each day, just waiting to get well. I needed to do more than eat oatmeal, and observe. Where prayer might point me in the right direction, I needed to participate. I began to focus my energy on unleashing my own natural healing abilities. I immediately corrected my own inner dialog and replaced "I feel like I'm dying" with: "I see myself healing and alive past 85." This seems a bit complicated for a mantra, but when I tried to say I'm well, I'm healthy, it didn't work, and it felt like a lie. So I replaced it instead with an honest vision that that I could work towards.

Moving on the new path of possibilities, my hope was further renewed when I recognized the conversation between my heart and my mind. That "feeling of doom," was the dialog. It helped me to visualize the harmony; my heart was communicating with my mind. What I needed was to capitalize on my own trusted source within me.

Notes from my heart:

What I know for sure, ten years later: In the aftermath of a heart attack you tend to examine both life and death differently. Somewhere in the recovery process you may develop a unique perspective or survival skill. Maybe you'll develop a greater appreciation of your time, or the gift of awareness. If used properly you'll reset your course, and create a lifetime series of joyful moments.

1. For me, the medication dulled my mental clarity, and prevented my ability to tap into my own natural healing resources. In return it temporarily halted my healing process. Work with your doctor to find the proper dosage for you. We all metabolize these drugs differently.

2. If your doctor is not cooperative in adjusting the medication for your well-being, find a new doctor. This is too important to your over-all recovery. Remember one half of women will die within the first year of a heart attack.

3. If you need inspiration for positive reinforcement, I recommend a trip to the library. Some of my favorite books are by Napoleon Hill and Norman Vincent Peale. If listening is more relaxing for you, most material can be found on tape or compact disk. Television offers a host of wonderful religious programming. I'm most inspired by TD Jakes, Joyce Meyers and Joel Osteen. And I look forward to the PBS (Public Broadcast System) wonderful specials with Dr. Wayne Dyer and Dr. Christiane Northrop.

4. Examine your inner dialog. What messages are you repeating to yourself on a daily basis? Is it healthy and positive reinforcement?

5. Examine your environment are you surrounded by people that are supportive and uplifting? Can you eliminate the relationships that tend to be energy drains or at least modify the amount of time you spend with them?

Chapter 8:
When the Going gets Tough

"We are like tea bags-we don't know our own strength until we're in hot water." —Sister Busche

Today more than ever we understand the power of positive thoughts and behavior. Its use is commonplace in business, religion and health care. Athletes' hone their skill to their highest potential with it. We elected a President because he presented a positive message and offered, hope. It appears we've exhausted the complicated and gone back to the basics. That's the success this country was built on, the heart of each ordinary individual.

Individuality has also surfaced in medical circles. There's a new acceptance in heart related medical treatment. No longer are woman and men treated with the same medications or certainty. The gold standard drugs for heart disease may not perform with gender equality. We all need to be treated independently. While it appears to be a baby step in comparison to the giant leap we need to prevent the loss of lives the first year after a heart attack. Gradually we may see a greater impact when the entire medical community adapts to, and adopts these changes.

There were then, and are today, many books outlining how to heal the physical heart. Each of these books offers a slightly different spin of the food pyramid, and the magic diet. All the books are complete with recipes, beneficial exercise routines, and recommendations for life style improvements. With the addition of proper sleep these established guidelines are vitality important. And many of us need medication as well. Sadly for some, it's more complicated and these best intended remedies don't always address the cause.

The care that includes the mind/body aspect is known today as Alternative, Holistic or Complementary. Integrative care is a combination of the Alternative and Traditional or Conventional medical care. Physicians that specialize in the Integrative care are difficult to find in most states. In Naturopathy there are two types of doctors the ND which is a Naturopath Doctor or a NMD a Naturopath Medical Doctor. Both focus their efforts on the cause of disease by understanding the body, mind, and spirit of the patient. They use a variety of methods as needed to support the body's own healing abilities.

And the new journey began…I arrived at the Complementary Care Clinic with renewed courage to fight-on and a good feeling about the process I was about to embark on. Almost eight months to the day of the heart attack, just two weeks after the latest three stent placement, and Brachytherapy. Although mentally improved, I was not well, and I was running out of options. I prayed so much I think God was tired of hearing from me.

After a ninety minute discussion, and thorough review of my medical history with the Director (an NMD) of the clinic, he determined I would be a good fit for their programs. He recommended that I begin with their Nutritionist and Pastoral Counseling. He said the counselors would introduce me to nutrition counseling, vitamin supplements, psychotherapy, meditation, yoga, guided imagery, massage and acupuncture. I guess you could say he threw the Homeopathic book at me. Then he gently placed his hands on mine and suggested, "Based on our conversation you've experienced a tremendous loss of family in a short period of time. The chronic level of grief and stress has taken a toll on your health. Love is… our relationships… our family. These are all matters of the heart."

I wasn't sure what to expect when I started with the clinic. But I wasn't disappointed. If nothing else the atmosphere that they create is comforting and empowering. The air is saturated with warm souls and positive energy. In spite of the mental grilling about my history, I left there with a sense of peace and accomplishment. I was convinced I finally found the right path. My only confusion was how I blend the two medical approaches. Conventional medicine saved my life on more than one occasion. I wouldn't want to go through strep throat without penicillin; the fevers almost killed me or deliver a baby without the best drugs. Then I asked myself is anyone demanding your loyalty to one or the other? While the two disciplines weren't in total agreement on how to achieve the desired outcome they were committed to best possible health for their patients.

During my car ride home, my thoughts were all over the place; *Hello God, did you hear him…he suggested that I have a broken heart. And I thought it was so complicated. He made it sound so easy. Great now I know. But how do I fix a broken heart? Sounds like a song. Can we put a rush on it.?" And her tombstone read; here lies a.... that ran out of... Oh stop it! Don't you go there! You are not ready to go anywhere...you went through all of this to live remember? Please God.*

It was just a few weeks past Christmas. I smiled as I remembered my presents. We had a theme that year. It wasn't choreographed, it just happened. Everyone bought me a heart. Maybe they knew? My husband bought me a heart shaped diamond ring. From my kids and grandchildren I received two necklaces with single hearts, a heart bracelet and a heart shaped pin. Like they say "great minds think alike," and we all had fun with it as I opened my gifts.

My health also changed the tone and depth of personal conversations. Everyone was more careful to say the things that are often left unsaid, just in case. I'm so grateful they did. Those words often served as my life line. I had so much to live for. If I learned anything from this time in my life, it's all about love. This is the one true "circle," the more love you give, the more you receive. Love is a consecrated spirit, with a sacred force.

I scheduled the follow up appointments quickly and started that week with the Nutritionist. After reviewing my recent health history she asked if I had been given a blood test for my level of: Lipoprotein-called, Lp- (a)-pronounced, "LP little a." "Not to my knowledge," I confessed. "You have six stents and no one has tested you for Lp- (a)? "What is it?" I asked.

"Lipoprotein (a) it's a genetic blood marker for early onset heart disease. It's a serious risk factor. In high levels it will cause the forming of scar tissue in the artery. Like stents for example; Lp- (a) will react to the new stent by trying to repair it. That's its job in normal levels, but in abnormal levels it will go into over drive repairing the artery and close it with the scar tissue, restenosis. There is nothing you could have done to prevent it. It's an inherited genetic weakness. It's very difficult to control," she explained. Lp-(a) is thought to regulate clot formation (thrombosis) and inhibit blood thinning, which can lead to blood circulation issues. There's also a problem in that it causes the blood to be sticky which potentially can cause the blood to clot more easily.

Well, I got the answers I prayed for. I knew the test results before they came back. My Lp- (a) was off the charts. And there too ends the mystery of the anomaly. I would expect that Kim had it too.

I went through a period of questioning everything, nothing appeared to be the way it was written, defined or should be. I had a heart attack when all of my life I had low blood pressure. I was constantly asked if I was diabetic. I wasn't. That was the one positive about the presence of the Lp-(a) I had one less thing to feel guilty about. There was nothing I could have done differently to prevent it; the Lp-(a). Amen. Had I known about it, there were many things I could have done to possibly prevent the heart attack. When they sent me for a stress test after my first stent closed, I passed it. I really had to convince my Cardiologist to listen to me. Most people would describe me as positive, cheerful, and laid back person. I love art; music and glorious aromas. I'm not a typical stressed out personality. With all of the recent hospital stays, why am I the only female on the Cardiac floor? And no one is anywhere near my age. I wasn't looking to socialize but it sure makes you wonder. The Cardiac floor was full with; older miserable men that fussed and complained all day long. Then you question the obvious, why are they alive, and my sister is dead? She had so much to live for. She was needed by so many. She was thin, active, rode bikes with the kids every day. She was the epitome of health and beauty in her satin lined casket. With so much emphasis placed on heart health and weight; the guys on the Cardiac floor were all skinny too. Maybe if they ate more they wouldn't be so darn crabby. They would begin their morning by badgering the nurses for their enemas. With two Cardiologists and an Internist involved in my care and don't forget the second opinion from a third Cardiologist in Chicago-a huge, well known, teaching hospital and I'm diagnosed with an inherited heart problem, found only by a Nutritionist. A broken heart and Lp- (a), I had a lot to sort out.

Notes from my heart:

What I now know ten years later: Make a conscious effort to have positive feelings flowing through you as much as possible. If you find joy in helping others, get out and spread that joy. Reach out to your loved ones and create special moments. Not just romantic moments, although those are extremely important if you have a significant other in your life. And can be a necessary reinforcement of your bond. But also time alone with family members; your son, daughter, grandchild, and parents. Go out to lunch, a play or a movie. That one on one time can replenish the soul.

1. You can't reach a goal that hasn't been set. Write down your goals. Every time you accomplish something new, celebrate it, take a breath and set a new goal.

2. Honestly, the thing that truly helped me endure the health crisis was when I decided to take vacations from our worries. We didn't go anywhere but for a few days at a time I refused to think about any problems, no "what ifs." What if this happens or what if that happens. I didn't allow myself to wonder when this would heal or that. The more of these mental vacations that I took; the better I coped with the everyday needs of our situation. Some might consider it another form of denial but for me it was truly a respite that allowed me to come back to my problems with a fresh perspective.

3. The Power-The more I prayed for guidance the more creative energy I found to solve problems. *The Bible*: Matthew 11:28-

"Come unto me all ye that labor and are heavy laden and I will give you rest."

4. Miracles-They won't happen if you don't expect them. Visualize yourself healed.

5. Choose your support system carefully; someone you wish to be part of it isn't always capable. People don't always handle illness well.

6. Choose people that share your core beliefs and that understand your spiritual needs, maybe someone that would pray with you, or for you.

Chapter 9:
Seven, the Number of Completion

"My life is my message." —Mahatma Ghandi

Have you ever been on a boat being rowed by a higher power? Throughout this storm, that's how I felt. Yet, I'd still ask from time to time, *"God is that really you?"* Then I'd review the reality of the situation; how many near death experiences do you need in a year before you declare yourself a survivor? And no matter how disturbing the news was-specifically in this case of the Lp-(a), the less fear I felt. I accepted the anomaly with a come on, bring it on attitude. My approach was; okay now you know, what's next? I just wanted the answers. Not just for me, but understanding its genetic component; I needed answers for about eight kids, mine and Kim's, and how about the next generation, my grandchildren. And when I remembered to follow the DNA trail to my three other living siblings, and their children, the potential magnitude of this problem was enormous. It was my job; I was the first, to survive it.

A speed boat might have been faster than a row boat, but that's not how these lessons are taught or unfold. No, the row boat would rock, and the water would splash me. But I had faith in the Captain not the vessel. Remember Jesus was born in a manger, a humble man. Who am I to complain? If the boat sprung a leak and if started to sink- just as miraculously- before I could sing the second verse of; "There's a hole in my bucket dear Liza dear Liza there's a hole in my bucket dear Liza a hole"…A patch would appear and a wave would stir-up yet another message in a bottle, floating conveniently alongside the boat. Just within my grasp… Quickly, I was back on course and gratefully humming, "row, row your boat gently down the stream"…

That time the message fell out of the heart book the hospital provided. It was the in notes I had taken, (the notes I had forgotten) about the Cardiologist that specialized in female heart issues. You know from the nurse with the under-ground information. She addressed certain subjects in whispers, shared secret formulas and swore me into her confidence. I wondered; does this kind of thing only happen to me? I'm sure not. Maybe I'm just more open to it. This is the material for a great novel, complete with spy quality. While it possess' the character of the under-ground, it was strangely delivered on Angels Wings.

If I were asked; who was one of the most important people in my life- you know, one of my top five. I would tell you about a man that I've never met. I was introduced only to his work, and his knowledge saved my life. Through prayer I found my most crucial source of information. It appeared in the nick of time as always, and arrived in the most unconventional, yet modern methods for that time. It came to me through an internet website, and subsequently a series of books he authored, that man is Dr. Stephen Sinatra. Today his specialty is Integrative Cardiology.

Ten years ago, the internet did not have a reputation for reliable information. I, too, was skeptical about getting heart information from an internet source, until I started to read his website. It was as though he knew me. He provided information on female heart attack symptoms, and nutritional support to improve your overall health. He shared patient stories, and outcomes. Guided women on what blood test to request from their Cardiologist, what the test results meant and what course of action to take. He even discussed Lp-(a) and developed a formula of vitamins to lower it. The best part was when he addressed a vitamin plan to take during recovery from angioplasty and stents. He understood the connection of heart ache and a broken heart. Sometime that year he published his book titled "*Heart Sense for Woman.*" I think I purchased one of the first copies. It became my heart instruction manual. I recommend it to any woman with heart disease issues-I've purchased many copies over the years-and have often given it to friends in heart trouble. With only one request, pass it on to someone in need, because when you need it, you may need it fast.

By the time my test results came back, regarding the level of my Lp-(a) I had a decent knowledge of it effects. I copied Dr. Sinatra's formula for lowering Lp-(a), and was prepared to discuss it with my Nutritionist on my next visit. She knew of his reputation and was willing to incorporate his suggestions into my recovery plan. She developed a complete daily plan for me including, what time of the day to take my medications. When I should snack, and when to take the vitamins-thankfully many of the same vitamins I needed for the Lp-(a) were also helpful with the after care for angioplasty and stent.

She explained the difference between them: some vitamins were fat soluble others were water soluble. She warned me that it might take weeks to feel the improvement but not to get discouraged, it would be noticeable and soon. That was something to look forward to.

The bond with the Pastoral Counselor-(Psychotherapist) was immediate. It took two sessions with her just to provide the information of my family tree and dynamics. There were and are many people in my daily circle. This was my first time in therapy. I was probably difficult to follow. She referred me immediately to the web site of Bella Ruth Naperstak and her guided imagery material, and walked me though guided imagery in her office. Together we addressed my most pressing issue-the potential of restenosis. I know I was given the latest cure with the Brachytherapy-but why did I feel terrible. Together we came up with the imagery. Popular at the time, was a game called, Pac-Man. The Pac-Man travel through a maze –I would visualize the maze, and the maze became my arteries. The Pac-Man would move through the arteries and swallow up anything foreign in their path-in my case scar tissue. Each night I'd play the guided imaginary tape for *"Heart Health"* (from the Naperstak collection) as I went to sleep, I would visualize the Pac-Men working as I slept. Always a fan of multi-tasking this concept was good for me, and provided plenty of laughs. Conversation about my health had become too heavy; this provided a light alternative…So when asked, "How are you feeling?" I would reply rather matter-of- fact, "Oh, I recently hired some Pac-Men to clean my arteries. Yeah, they're my night crew- they work as I sleep." It allowed for a good laugh on a tough subject. I introduced guided imagery to anyone that would listen to me.

The blessings abound; my Complementary Care team understood the seriousness of my condition and moved quickly to expose and teach me methods to renew my health. We were creating an environment for me to heal, a constant spiritual and Holistic flow of intravenous feedings that sent messages to my mind/body.

It was the beginning of March 2001, ten months after the heart attack, two months after the Brachytherapy and stents. After a good night's rest with my Pac-Man guided imagery, I woke, did some of my morning yoga exercise, followed by prayer and meditation. This was my new morning ritual. I tried to ignore-"*It*" for a couple of days, but denial was more difficult when I was in touch with my emotions and spiritually connected. "*It* "was the feeling of doom, and "It" was back. Finally, I surrendered to the thought and the feeling, as I knelt on the floor in prayer. And I sobbed. I was completely confused and frustrated. Was the last ten months a series of fruitless exercises? Was I supposed to die? Had I somehow cheated death? I searched for the purpose and the meaning. What benefit did these last months of my life serve? Did I somehow advance science? How many more stents can you have before they refer to your heart as bionic? Was another stent even a possibility? *Oh God... what's this all about?*

That life boat must have come by, you know that row boat, and it found me curled up in bed, in a fetal position. In spite of all of my recent efforts, I was more than mentally exhausted, I was a wreck. When the doom came back it almost stole my hope. A couple of hours had passed; I must have gone through many different scenarios in my mind. But finally I sat up regained my composure and said,

"Put up your dukes woman and fight. You have so much to live for". The "put up your dukes" was a line my Dad often used when he'd play fight with my son's. I think it's a line from an old John Wayne movie. Maybe in my time of trouble Dad was there with me, whispering, "Get up Pam, and don't give up." He had been dead about ten years at that point. During my crisis I missed him terribly.

I pulled myself out of bed and called my Cardiologist. He scheduled me for the Cardiac Catherization Lab early the next morning. "You know the routine," he said, "Go directly to the Emergency Room if you need to, Do Not Wait." Then I called my husband, I asked him not to tell the kids this time. "We'll just tell them that I have an early morning meeting. We'll be out of the house before they wake-up. Please Chris they will be so frightened-they thought the Brachytherapy was the final procedure." "So did I," he said sadly, "So did I."

Climbing back on the row boat was easier this time; a sense of peace welcomed me as I reached my spot. Of course I requested my usual assurances, "God...?" I had just celebrated my 47th birthday the week before. My oldest granddaughter's birthday was the next day. I always prepared for surgery with a vision of what was coming next, the next celebrations, the next family event. And I visualized myself there, at her 4th birthday party, a warm embrace, with kisses on her beautiful, dimpled cheek, and a wink. Why a wink, it was our thing; from an early age before she could speak I'd wink at her and she'd wink back. It was so darn adorable. These wonderful relationships and celebrations carried me through each crisis.

In the Cardiac Catherization Lab I updated my Cardiologist on my guided imagery efforts, he listened politely. "It's important," I said, "that you keep me awake as long as possible because I need to get a really good look at my physical heart for visualization purposes." I don't recall him agreeing and at one point, as usual, he asked if I was having heart pain and I said, "Yes, as I told you I haven't felt right since they placed those three stents." That ended the visualization, he put me to sleep. I woke up to my Cardiologist and my husband arguing above me. My husband wanted me to have a coronary artery by-pass, open heart surgery. My Cardiologist said it was not necessary, she's too young; you don't want that for her. "Those only last ten years," he said. The back and forth between them went on for a few minutes. Somewhere in their conversation I realized I received stent #7 and the tears flowed. That put an immediate halt to their fighting. My Cardiologist then calmly drew a picture of an artery on his clip board and as he drew he said, "I have good news, Pam there was no scar tissue this time." And he then very carefully worded his findings; "The problem was a bend in the artery caused by the concentration of stents in-this-one area. To correct it, I placed a stent further down the artery to stabilize it. This should work." He squeezed my hand and said, "I promised I wouldn't let anything happen to you. You're going to be okay." From the moment I woke up from the Brachytherapy I questioned the three stents his colleague placed that day. It was one of those moments-when you hear "red flag- listen up- something's not right." Whether you feel it in your gut or hear it in your head you've learned to trust it, because time will always prove its accuracy. I don't think my Cardiologist was pleased either from his reaction, but I think we just hoped his colleague knew something we didn't. Well that was my prayer. Once the stents are placed, it's done. They don't come back out.

Bible scholars have found what they believe to be significant connections with certain numbers and the way they are used in the text. For instance the number eight is considered the number of new beginnings. The number seven is God's perfection or completeness. Oh I hope so. And I row, row, row, the boat gently...

Notes from my heart:

What I know for sure, ten years later: Even coping and recovering from a health crisis needs good time management. We created my own cardiac rehab, with a Holistic approach. Achieving success was all in Pam's plan ...

1. My original care plan consisted of nutrition/vitamin counseling. Pastoral counseling: psychotherapy, hypnosis and in those sessions, I was taught guided imagery, and meditation practices. At least once a week I had a choice of massage therapies. I also engaged in the classes they offered; therapeutic yoga, and Tai Chi.

2. I planned and posted my daily schedule including exercise time and weekly appointments.

3. I had meal plans with a grocery list of pantry staples to stay on course with nutrition plan.

4. I charted medications and vitamins.

5. I started journaling to aid in unscrambling my thoughts and combined it with a gratitude journal. It was always easier to think of things I was grateful for.

6. It was highly recommended that I learn how to sleep for at least eight hours each night. For years I was surviving on five or six. With the removal of caffeine from my diet, and daily exercise I was able to retrain myself in about a month or so.

7. My Care Team recommended that I track my blood pressure. I purchased my own monitor. Knowing my heart rate and blood pressure numbers was so important. It helped me to understand the affects I was feeling when my blood pressure was very low. It also provided a record I needed to discuss with my Cardiologist of the impact the medication was having on me. For people that suffer from high blood pressure it's also imperative to know; because of the association of stroke and kidney disease. To get accurate readings, do the following:

- No talking or fidgeting it can throw off a blood pressure reading.

- Blood pressure can be influenced by movement or anxiety, sit quietly for a few minutes before taking a reading.

- Get the right cuff size for your arm. One that is too small or too large will give false readings.

- Take readings on both arms. Some people have considerable differences in blood pressure between their two arms.

- Take a reading; wait; take another. One blood pressure measurement may not be accurate. So get at least two readings, several minutes apart, and average them.

- Make sure arms and feet are well-positioned. Improper body, arm and leg position can falsify blood pressure readings.

- To follow the guidelines and get the most accurate results, you should sit comfortably in a backrest chair with your feet flat on the floor.

Chapter 10:
Have Mercy

"The unexamined life is not worth living." —Socrates

Each time I went back to work after one of the stent procedures the whole concept made less and less sense to me. I kept dragging myself back to work, did the best I could and always felt lousy. My motivation was to provide normalcy for all the people that depended on me. Returning to work suggested to all involved that I was better. But I wasn't. It was time to stop perpetuating the same cycle. Enough! Three weeks after the procedure for stent #7, on April 13, 2001, I gave a respectable notice and resigned from my position as a Hotel General Manager. At one time, I enjoyed the job. I was successful at it, and I truly cared about my team there. Every morning during my illness, they held a prayer circle and prayed for my health and recovery. It was very difficult to leave them, I felt as though I was betraying them. But I longed for rest and time to heal. That wasn't possible with the schedule I kept. Life had moved me in a different direction that year. When I asked myself what I liked or wanted to do with my life, that job was no longer a priority.

Personally, and under the counsel of my Complementary Care team I started to look forward to having the time to restore my body, and mind. Time is a luxury today for most women and for the first time in my life I was in a financial position to consider it. Imagine, finally having time to think about, and pursue what my heart desired.

My decision found wings and was expedited when my husband was offered his dream job around the same time. Everything pointed towards change and a move. *So God... Pennsylvania?*

On May 23, 2001, a very proud teary eyed mom, watched her beautiful, intelligent daughter receive her college diploma. Now it was official-she is a teacher. From the time she was a toddler she'd line up all her dolls and stuffed animals and hold class.

One year to the day of my heart attack-surrounded by the loudest bunch on the bleachers, there was my family, whistling, whooping and hollering for their sister. My husband led the event. They make everything fun, I thought. *"God I love these guys."* What a proud moment, and thanks to the power of suggestion and an empty wallet, she was able to accomplish it in four years.

Naturally on my anniversary day, it was time to re-examine the difficult year gone by. During this annual inventory, I realized that something was different. Could it be-I was healing. As I expected, through my heart/soul whispers, I knew the restenosis was over.-With a whoosh it was out of my life. It's hard to describe, calm replaced the anxiety. I guess the #7 was my number of completion. For me this was a day of gratitude, celebration and reflection.

But at the end of the day, I remained painfully aware of the frightening female statistic: that half of women that experience heart attacks will die within a year. Yes indeed I had that knowledge even ten years ago. I discovered it, as I researched Lp-(a), the combination left me trembling. Armed with this knowledge declaring victory would have been premature. Although I recognized the progress, I was still extremely fragile mentally and physically from my year of procedures.

Therapy provided me the opportunity to release feelings of guilt for not being able to accomplish everything. My root was bonded in the spiritual, my sixth sense, and that was my reality. If I wanted restoration in my body I knew I had to be healed in the spirit. Until I was able to release myself from self-imposed obligations and burdens my physical body struggled to heal. For me therapy was equally as important as any medicine or vitamins I swallowed.

It has taken many years to find the right words to define these periods of utter chaos in my life; the storms. These periods of growth and change that sometimes make you feel like you're under assault; for instance when lightning hits your house or the kids suffer simultaneously from temporary diminished capacity. My Mom would refer to these days as running between a sweat and a tear; when we would go from one sick relative to another, appliances breaking, and pipes leaking. Whether you view these times of trouble as misaligned planets or products of a full moon, it happens to the best of us. We're all students of crisis management, that's life. Today, ten years later, enjoying a higher realm of wisdom, when it's all swirling around me, I simply laugh and say, "The Angels are tickling me." Because I know, by using prayer as my response to life problems, it's always available to me and I'm strengthened by it. This too, is no perfect science; as life can leave me speechless and or angry at times. But I hold on tight and pray for the stillness. I'm a work in progress. And, I do wish every word or thought out my mouth was peacefully composed. But they're not. I'm all too human, and likely to say things like, *"God you're kidding me right? I heard about that sense of humor of yours."* I believe my path is guided by God. As I grow in faith I find myself apologizing less often for my cynical thoughts and remarks.

The graduation would be our last celebration in that house. When I placed the house on the market it sold in three days. We would be leaving Maryland for Pennsylvania. We had already purchased a new home, still in close proximity to our kids allowed me to easily surrender to another move. All the kids would be within an hour's drive, our two daughters and granddaughter chose to stay with us. After our family visitors left we would begin packing and move the following weekend, never a dull moment.

Our new home was set slightly higher than the homes in this lovely upscale neighborhood. It was surrounded by a variety of old gorgeous trees, all in full bloom for our arrival that June 2001. We were greeted by a breath taking view. From our yard you couldn't see the neighbor's houses, which led to a feeling of peaceful seclusion. The first night in the new house I slept twelve hours straight. When I woke, I couldn't hear a sound, and the room was dark except for the light that caught my eye under the bathroom door. It was from the skylight over the Jacuzzi garden tub…So cool. When I checked my clock it said it was noon, it must be wrong. When I opened the blinds the sun was shining and when I opened the French doors to the adjacent deck the birds were gloriously singing. Welcome home.

Could it be- my new bedroom was sound proof-get out town! Oh it gets better, at least twice a day I'd swim in my large "in ground" heated pool at the temperature I desired- WARM. I loved to swim at night, and float on my back staring up at the evening sky and the glistening stars-then I'd pitch myself to see if it was real-*God am I here on Earth or did you take me to Heaven?*

I continued with my daily ritual of yoga, meditation and prayer. At night I fell asleep to guided imagery. I also kept my appointments in Maryland with my Care Team-it was only an hour ride, heck where else would I drive my new car-with the cool sun roof and the awesome stereo system. I'd always try to meet one of the kids after my appointment for lunch if they were available. They claimed they could hear me coming from the music blaring in my car. - "Oh yeah, Patti Labelle or Aretha Franklin-here comes Mom." Was I having a mid life crisis, or just glad to be alive-probably both, I do know I was tired of always driving the lesser car because I didn't have as far to drive. My cars always got passed down to the kids so I made sure they were safe and economical. In this walking on the wild side phase- I would grocery shop and not plan the meals based on what was on sale. I would shop (sometimes) at the gourmet grocery store and cook it in my gourmet kitchen complete with a Jenn-Air grill. The acceptance of that second class citizen mentality left me around stent #7. Scrimping and saving and doing everything myself expired, I had a "Don't do list" considerably longer than- No snow shoveling.

Notes from my heart:

What I know for sure, ten years later: We all need to be touched. The therapeutic benefits of massage, reflexology, and acupressure are curative.

1. Massage therapy is considered an Alternative or Holistic therapy. It was derived and practiced for centuries in countries around the world. Many massage therapies are very similar with name variations.

2. Today, massage is big business. There are literally hundreds to choose from. In the United States the therapists are certified and often work in conjunction with hospitals, Alternative, Holistic, Complementary Care Clinics and popular day spas.

3. Their health benefits are widely accepted. They're known to improve circulation, and promote healing. The sessions are generally 30 to 60 minutes in length.

4. It is generally not covered by health insurance and can be too costly for many. You and/or a partner can rent, purchase massage videos or take a class to learn the basic techniques. Your local library would be a good and free source.

5. Create a healing space in your home. For the cost of an hour massage you can purchase a massage cushion that you attach to your favorite chair as well as a foot massager. With a one-time larger investment you can purchase a massage chair. With the addition of music, meditation or guided imaginary CD's you've created a restorative setting.

6. Consult your doctor before engaging in massage therapy; deep muscle massage is not recommended for some individuals with cardiovascular or vascular health issues.

7. Swedish massage is probably the most common, with massage oils or lotion. The strokes vary from circular motions to long smooth strokes. I found it to be very gentle and relaxing.

8. An aromatherapy massage: is usually the Swedish massage with one or more essential oils to address specific needs. Select plant oils with options from energizing, stress reducing to calming.

9. Reiki therapy vs. Touch therapy: The word "Reiki" in Japanese translates roughly as "universal life force energy." The Reiki procedure works something like this: the Reiki master holds their hands over your fully clothed body - and uses their spiritual energy to administer the healing treatment. This channeling of good energy will then encourage the patient to heal. The practitioner never makes contact with the patient's skin. The environment is totally relaxed, and candle light; soothing music and aromatherapy are used to put the client in a totally relaxed state.

10. Shiatsu: is the traditional therapeutic form of massage using deep penetrating pressure to stimulate acupressure points, the same points used in acupuncture. Releasing these healing points opens the channels of energy and blood circulation to

nourish the internal organs, glands, muscles, nerves, and vital centers of the body.

11. Reflexology: Reflexology points on the hands and feet stimulate the nerve endings, which send healing messages to all parts of the body via neurological pathways.

12. Acupressure: Acupressure points have similar benefits, which stem from balancing the body's life energy through a system of meridian pathways.

13. When Reflexology and Acupressure are used together, the energy released joins forces to heal the body, thus increases the effectiveness of results. The integration of Reflexology and Acupressure therapy creates a more efficient, Holistic healing practice.

*These are therapeutic choices I have used; I enjoyed and received restorative benefits from all of them. There are still hundreds of options available. While I understand acupuncture has amazing results, I haven't attempted it yet. I perform reflexology and some acupressure remedies to my hands and feet to ease my recent arthritis pain. I have also invested in my own healing space complete with aromatherapy; actually I prefer it, because it's there when I need it.

Chapter 11:
Therapy

"The great awareness comes slowly piece by piece. The path of spiritual growth is a path of lifelong learning."
  —Elisabeth Kubler-Ross

Therapy was working for me; it was my panacea. Each session helped me to unscramble my thoughts. For forty five minutes once a week I would greet my therapist, sit down and talk. When I started to talk, I realized how much of my adult life was formed by action or reaction to whatever crossed my path. My secrets were revealed in that room. Oh, don't get excited there were no sins committed, I didn't have time. Unfortunately, that was the secret. I was very much a part of a generation of woman that advanced our female rights. I remember holding my first management position in the restaurant industry in the mid 1970's. When a food delivery would come in I'd be chasing the driver to sign off on the order as he'd be looking for the male manager. When I told him I was the manager he'd ask if I was the owner's daughter or *something*. We all knew what the inference to, *something*, was.

As I transitioned into the hotel industry in the 1980's there were only a handful of woman in the General Managers position countrywide. I was an example, a voice, and the role model for other woman and I knew it. While I can't say it was something I aspired to, as it was for some woman, when I found myself caught up in it, I accepted my responsibility with a serious effort. What should have been my greatest compliment is when I would ask other women I coached or mentored what they saw themselves doing in five to ten years. Their reply was, "I want to be just like you." Everything inside me was screaming "No Don't" but, I'd smile with the understanding it was meant as a compliment and hoped their road would be easier. Quite possibly it was. As time passed discrimination laws were advanced, sexual harassment was addressed in the work place, and I can't speak for all women but I know my wage was fair. One of the greatest gifts was the Family Leave Act. While it came a little too late for me, it made for a less hostile environment for all, men and women alike. It gave us permission to focus energy on our family. Everyone needed time to take our kids to the dentist or an hour off for a school event.

That's the big secret. The advancement of woman didn't come without a cost, women were exhausted. There were few role models for us. As a whole we were over-committed and our lives became quite complicated. The best of us would try harder and harder to organize all the details of our existence but, while best case scenarios may have gotten the job done, it did nothing to protect us from our self neglect. We were encouraged by some, and envied by many. The commercial media portrayed us as glamorous. And they cleverly sold a fortune in products that supported our multi-tasking adventures. While appearing amazingly beautiful we cooked, did laundry and cleaned after working all day. We were driven by the Supermom Syndrome we created.

On a positive note, we no longer had to hide a pregnancy for fear of being fired or losing our jobs while on medical leave. However, there were also many unpleasant aspects. For instance, watching a new mom come back to work and cry most of the day at her desk with separation anxiety from her new infant. Puppies get more time with their mothers then some babies did. Or the phone tie ups at 3:00 each afternoon as the latch key kids called in. There were problems from sleep deprivation to trustworthy day care systems. I guess someone had to go first to create the options and the more family friendly environment we have today. But it wasn't without cost and it's not a coincidence that female heart disease soared during this period.

I never pushed for a promotion because in the hotel industry the majority of higher positions meant travel. I didn't feel you could have two traveling parents-I was even afraid to take a vacation from the "Brainy Bunch." Twice a year I had to travel for mandatory company meetings and in my absence, just a few days always ended in an unpleasant story.

Really at the end of the day I wasn't as ambitious as my husband. My priority was to provide a loving, safe and harmonious home life for my family. And my desire was to create a positive work environment where-by our employees could grow and prosper while increasing company profits. I wanted success in both areas, and it was a challenge.

It's too bad that The Center of Disease Control didn't identify Super-Mom Syndrome as a contagious disease that went rampant in the 1980's and slap a warning label on some of us- Warning: Code Level Red: This group is a Hurricane in High Heels. Performing at extreme stress levels for an extended period of time may lead to serious illness.

During therapy you deep clean your closets. It's where you can tell your secrets. A place where we can say, we don't always enjoy every aspect of our life, without judgment. And that's another secret, because life was not fair in our homes either; each day we're doing more than what was expected of our male counterparts. Many of us held an underlying anger. Whether fueled from heavy burdens, frustration, stress levels, or exhaustion this group cried secret tears.

It took two years to sort through almost fifty years. I discovered my chronic level of stress didn't begin in adulthood. It began during childhood. I don't know how you prepare for life without some dysfunctional element in childhood. By embracing that theory I wasn't disappointed. I'm willing to say, my childhood prepared me well. I had developed pretty good coping skills. And was able to identify through therapy, the self preservation techniques I acquired along the way. However, this Supermom should have sought help sooner. The trauma of the seven years of loss was one brick too many on my existing load.

As I unscrambled, I grew in confidence that I indeed still had a future to prepare for, and a purpose. As cliché as it sounds; I rediscovered myself. Going forward I chose my hats carefully. For most of my life I didn't feel I had options. I did what was necessary to provide for my family. As a divorced-single mother I worked evenings for the least amount of time away from my son's wake time. When they started school I switched hours. Each job or career choice had to provide me the ability to best care for my family.

When I married my husband, his career took precedence, and as such was the reason for eight moves in a twenty year period. A huge cause of stress, I had to be the source of the calm and stability during each move, the protector of all the necessary records for easy school transition.

The frazzled mother that ran from soccer, to baseball fields after work in high heels. (There was no such thing as business casual.) I'm sure you saw me; the lady that could pull shin guards out of her purse or a jock strap out of her brief case and carry the team drinks in an ice chest on her hip. Yeah, that nut was me. Once in a while I'd luck out and have three kids playing in the same park on different fields. Then my biggest challenge was to remember the supportive lingo, "Hey there great job goalie!" -shouldn't be said to a short stop. Not and unless you want your kid to turn purple and pass out from embarrassment. Usually I'd follow the lead of another parent. Until I was told more than once by the kids, I was cheering for the wrong team.

Obviously, I didn't play sports as a kid. The closest I got to sports was my Dad watching the Cubs in the kitchen and my brother watching the White Sox in the family room.

I loved it when my husband was in town. And when my oldest son got his license, I rejoiced, I had another driver. Just about the time I burnt him out, his younger brother got his license.

My husband was rarely there on the moving days he'd be in yet another town giving a presentation or something. It was customary for the flower truck to arrive about the same time the moving van did. The flower delivery was complete with an apology and thank you note, signed "Always and Forever, Chris." Our always and forever's came up for renegotiation each time we moved. I was generally resistant to the move for a multitude of reasons; the kids were in a great school system, I liked my job, etc. However and in hind sight I believe we were meant to be in those states and towns when we were, fate played a role in each move. There were people we were supposed to meet along the way. As hard as I fought, when it was our destiny, all the pieces would come together and I would be forced to surrender. Thankfully, our kids always fared well. They were provided many opportunities to be exposed to different cultures and learned to adapt to new situations. As a whole they were resilient. Sometimes they were excited about the new adventure; some were just happy to throw their stuff in a box rather than clean their bedroom. If it took a couple of weeks to find new friends, in the interim they always had each other. We had a 'moving mercy' upon us.

In therapy after you soul search for awhile, your target changes to those you surround yourself with. And you examine those relationships as well. Somewhere in therapy a flood of animosity came through about all the time I spent without my husband. So one day I said to my husband, "When do you think you'll be able to travel less? You know one day the kids are going to be gone and I don't want to be alone all the time." He made the serious mistake of joking about it, and replied, "Honey you get the kids out of the house and I'll come home." It was cleansing to finally bring these issues to the surface. I think I knew it when I saw my therapist feverishly taking notes like we had some major breakthrough, and quickly responding with "um hum, um hum, I see." Her reaction encouraged me to see that; yes, I had a long list of buried complaints. Then the flood gate opened-and I was as mad as hell that he wasn't with me when my Dad died, or my sister, and the day of my heart attack, I asked him not to leave, and he did anyway. But I didn't want to divorce him, maybe torture him for awhile.

No, therapy for me was going to take longer than anticipated because divorce was not my solution, not this time. I really wanted more of him, not less. I had developed a deep anger and resentment. I needed to find forgiveness.

As I unscrambled all these years, I only remembered being alone. I forgot, sometimes, there were reasons. He stayed home that weekend my Dad was dying, due to my insistence.-Dad was home in Chicago and we lived in Virginia at the time. It was our son's birthday; we planned a children's birthday party for him. I didn't want to disappoint our son. Dad died during the party that Sunday after-noon. After the party, Chris drove all night in a snow storm, with a car full of kids to be with me. Times were lean; we couldn't afford the huge expense of last minute tickets. Chris loved my Dad. My Dad became Chris' surrogate father when we met, his father died when he was only 15 years old. My Dad loved Chris too, and the two men were buddies. Unfortunately they bonded as drinking buddies, as well. I remember Dad saying to me the next morning after the two tied one on, "You need to watch him he may have a drinking problem," and I responded with "Gee Dad that's exactly what I was worried about last night when he helped you into bed."My Dad was a man of very few, carefully chosen words, unless he was drinking. This permitted my husband to have access to the unguarded side of his buddy. Chris had great insight into the great man that I called Dad, and he portrayed him perfectly. He was able to write and present a beautiful eulogy. I told him afterwards that I renewed his contract, he had ten more years.

Therapy taught me a lot about myself that I didn't realize. As I searched for forgiveness I realized I couldn't blame him for what I was lousy at. Always short of time, I made many concessions. I was managing my life by trying to limit the disappointment of others. Rather than rescheduling the birthday party I opted to not disappoint our son. My husband should have been with me and with my Dad. The more I moved over and made adjustments, the more danger I was in of falling off the cliff. More and more of me disappeared as my needs were rarely addressed.

Chris had the gift of selfishness, for self preservation. I resented him for having tunnel vision; if he needed to go to the gym, or for find time to play basketball during his 48 hour weekend visit, he'd take care of his needs first. I resented the amazing way he could tune out all the background chatter to hear the Bulls, Bears, Cubs, White Sox and Black Hawks. Oh yeah... he never missed a game on the weekends. We had satellite where ever we lived. It was part of the trinity of truck arrivals when we'd move: the moving, satellite, and the flower trucks.

In time I was able to accept yet another of our differences, however, I was left with what I felt were his misaligned priorities. Once in awhile I wished he would have postponed a meeting, sent someone from his team instead, or used a conference call method, rather than the reverse of trying to manage home/life events by phone. Not and until my therapy sessions forced us to communicate, is when we discovered that the corporate culture at the time was not family friendly either. Chris didn't feel he could manage it any other way. We each tolerated things we were not happy with because we were both driven by traditional values. He felt his responsibility was providing financially for his family. Even worse, his self worth is tied directly to his work. With few complaints he was completely supported by my efforts. He was virtually free of the hundreds of details it took to manage our large family. We both internalized any guilt, insecurity or unhappiness and pushed forward for the sake of our family.

The problem was we had no point of reference. We made it up as we went along. The portrait of the perfect family, we were envied and admired by many. It was the beginning of our generation's transformation of the workplace. However we were a bit different with five kids, two careers, and one parent often traveling. And still the kids were encouraged to be well rounded, with all the extracurricular activities of music, religion classes, dance and all the sports. We wanted it all and I refused to lower our family standards, I insisted we have dinner together. A Saint of a Mother, one would think. I'd cook all day on Sunday to prepare meals that we would heat up during the week. We hired no help, no cleaning service, no lawn help, and no laundry service. I believed everyone should have chores and learn responsibility. Do you have any idea how hard it is to teach this? I'm justified only by the fact that we've raised five terrific kids and my three sons are not only hands-on fathers they are terrific partners. They help with all the domestic duties at home. I'm proud of the changes we witness today. Family life, though still difficult, is more balanced with this current generation. But here too, someone had to go first, and do it wrong, before it was improved. And women have more options today than ever, I love that.

With each anniversary my husband jokingly asks for a renewal option. We've been together over 30 years today. We've always valued each other, and are mindful to be married one day at a time. I've heard couples of long marriages say their marriage endured the test of time because they never stopped loving each other at the same time. Love wasn't an issue for us, but as I worked through therapy our friendship was tested, he dreaded the days I had therapy. He never knew what memory from our past would come back and ambush him.

Our daughter-in-law went on and on one day complaining to me about her husband, (oh gosh my son) and as mother-in-laws go, I think I handled it pretty well. I asked her if he could still make her smile. She thought for a minute and said, "Yes smile… and laugh." "That's a pretty good start." I replied, "Marriage is hard, it takes work. I'm not criticizing divorce, I've been to the point of no return with someone and generally you're not smiling or laughing." That was ten years ago they're still together through the floods and tornadoes. I'm reminded the word "Love, is a verb-an action word, and it requires energy to nourish and preserve it.

Maybe some days you keep working at it because of the kids. We love all the same people. Hopefully, as in our case, you celebrate each other more often than tolerate each other.

If you asked me throughout the two years of therapy to draw my perfect husband it wouldn't resemble Chris, but ask me to draw my perfect man, you'd find my husband. I'd choose that man every time.

Notes from my heart:

What I know for sure, ten years later: Women have a tendency to internalize the big stuff. And my big stuff was a heavy burden on my soul. Psychotherapy was the foundation of my cure.

1. A good rapport with your therapist is critical. Choose a therapist with whom you feel comfortable expressing yourself with. Eventually when a bond or trust is developed; most of your secrets will be shared with this person.

2. You may be able to determine this on the telephone interview. However, the first appointment should be treated as a mutual interview during which both client and therapist decide whether or not a good working relationship is likely to form. You should present this suggestion to the therapist before the first appointment. This is a service you're paying for; don't be afraid to set the ground rules.

3. Type of questions to ask: Are you a licensed therapist?

4. How long have you been practicing? What are your areas of specialty? What kind of treatment do you usually use, and why do you feel this would be effective for my situation?

5. How long would you expect my treatment to last?

6. What are your fees? Will you accept my insurance?

7. And once you get all that out of the way; ask the real questions. The things your mind would be curious about it.

Where did they attend school, their curriculum vitae? Are the married? Where did they grow up? Do they have children? Ask them to tell you about themselves. I want to know about the person I share my time with. I need to, feel: a glimpse of their spirit, see: if they smile easily and touch: a hand shake. If you encounter a therapist that is resistant to answering reasonable questions, consider moving on.

8. Psychotherapy should not be a mystery, set goals and expectations. I had two goals when I started, first was to get unscrambled and the second was to find peace again.

9. If psychotherapy is not financially attainable, group sessions might be a less expensive option. Some counties offer mental health services on a sliding scale based on your income as do many religious based organizations.

10. The goal is self expression and the release of repressed emotions. Possibly you can achieve the same end goal with a different therapy, art, writing or a trusted friend that will commit to your process of healing.

Chapter 12:

From a Broken Heart to an Open Heart

"The secret of health for both mind and body is not to mourn for the past, worry about the future, or anticipate troubles but to live in the present moment wisely and earnestly."
    —Buddha

Clearly, I used each upcoming celebration for visualization purposes; it was my short term goal- just to be there. With modification, I used it for longer term goals too, for instance our son's wedding. I set healing milestones. I needed to achieve certain levels of wellness by September 15th. And I did, by the end of the first summer in the new house I was a physically stronger and had more energy. The timing was perfect; I would dance at their wedding, for hours if I so desired. I was walking further without the dread of exhaustion. The mind/body is resilient. As the memories of that time faded the more whole I felt. I'm sure all the swimming I did that summer contributed to my wellbeing. However, as we were preparing for the big day...

Tragedy struck our Nation on the morning of September 11, 2001; a World watched in disbelief the events of that day. Our family experienced moments of panic as we realized Chris was driving to upstate New York that morning, from the time he left he should have been in or near the city. From the television coverage we had no way to tell how far reaching the flames or the smoke was. But thank you God he answered his cell phone on the first ring; he was actually exiting the bypass around the city when I called, and was oblivious to the horror just a few miles from him. He said he heard what we were saying to him and then listened to the radio coverage, but not until he arrived at his destination and viewed the television coverage did he feel the complete impact of the tragedy. Those images…

My brave Chicago relatives were on the first permitted flights after 9/11, the wedding was just days later, as the airports reopened. Both elderly grandmothers-(our wedding warriors) made their way through hours of security for their grandson. They arrived at the wedding with moments to spare. It was a lovely wedding/reception and well attended considering the circumstances. While everyone put on their best face for the happy couple there was an undeniable air of uncertainty in the country.

I recognized pretty quickly that the stress of the 9/11 events was more than my fragile sponge for sadness or injustice could manage. I prayed daily for the families and limited my television coverage. I had to learn to protect myself.

As I recovered and eliminated health issues, there were serious realities I had yet to contend with. Were all my efforts actually healing my broken heart and what about the Lp-(a)? Was there any way for me to eliminate the vulnerability of another heart attack lurking around the corner?

What do you do when you're told you have an incurable problem? – This Lp-(a)? I went in search for answers and having time permitted the transference of energies. The time that I once spent at work, I used to try experimental treatments and to educate myself about Lp-(a). It became my full time job for awhile. My goal was to have a treatment plan for any family members that might inherit the Lp-(a).

I've mentioned that in retrospect each of our moves had a purpose. There were people we were meant to meet along the way. For my husband they were exciting career advancements. For me, I can associate each location with a specific time in my life. This move was an answer to my prayer for a place to heal. Our home provided a postcard setting that had a soothing energy surrounding it. With the heated pool, the Jacuzzi tub, and a hot tub attached to the pool, I had my own resort. I spent my days moving from one pleasure to another.

It's difficult to explain this presence of thought, other than to say I knew there was someplace I was to go, to heal there, and to return to wholeness. As my health improved I became braver and tried more controversial treatments to eradicate the Lp-(a). In support of another perfectly orchestrated plan; a couple of miles from the house there was an Alternative Care Clinic conveniently located that offered intravenous Chelation Therapy. Maybe I'd find the magic potent there.

Chelation Therapy is a treatment to restore blood flow and to eliminate toxins and heavy metals from your system. It involves the intravenous infusion of a prescription medicine called Ethylene Diamine Tetra-Acetic Acid (EDTA), plus vitamins and minerals at therapeutic dosages. The Chelation infusions are administered by slow drip, circulating through the blood stream treating the entire arterial system removing undesirable metals from the body. It was a time consuming process, I would meditate and use guided imagery during the hours of infusions. After fifty some treatments it again only lowered the Lp-(a) a couple of points and I couldn't be sure if it was the Chelation or the intense vitamin therapy. However, I did feel improvement.

There was also the discovery that during autopsy patients with heart disease were found to have levels of Chlamydia Pneumoniae in their diseased arteries. Not to be confused with the sexually transmitted disease, this type of Chlamydia is air borne. I was tested and of course had high levels of that too. I agreed to months of antibiotic therapy in hopes of possibly discovering a cure for both. The results were the same regarding Lp-(a). I continued to only move it a few points back and forth, and I haven't achieved a near normal level with all my efforts. But again I felt an overall health improvement. I know the repetition of this statement of feeling better or improved might be confusing, but I had accepted such a compromised feeling of poor health for so long it took a while to accept I could be better, and even better than that.

The Chelation followed by the antibiotic treatments was completed in a one year timeframe. I was reaching completion with the Alternative Clinic when there was yet another discovery of a danger-ous bacterium that's common to many illnesses; Nanobacteria. Nanoparticles are implicated in the harmful calcification associated with heart disease. The treatment at the time and in use today is EDTA and the antibiotic Tetracycline. I was feeling better than I had felt in years; I chose not to be tested for the Nanobacteria. The cure if necessary was a similar road to the one I had just traveled, with a different course of antibiotics, in my spirit I knew it was time to move on.

Throughout this year I also continued with my therapies in Maryland. Finally I ran out of things to talk about. My psychotherapy goal was to unscramble and find peace again. I achieved both, my thoughts were crystal clear. Especially after participating in some of the group sessions with other woman, and listening to what they perceived as problems. This confirmed my belief that I was coping well.

Finally I embraced Lp-(a). It's a part of me, and I hope that one day I will understand the purpose. I've changed the way I look at it over the years. I remain current on any new advances; I'm in process of trying an updated vitamin therapy. Although for the most part, I don't dwell on it. I remain committed to acquiring any and all knowledge for my family. I keep my blood thin with an aspirin regimen and slippery with fish oils and other vitamins. Three other members of my family currently have elevated levels of Lp-(a). While at this time it doesn't appear that we can avoid the heart disease, with proper intervention my hope is to eliminate the possibility of a heart attack.

For ten years, the best resource I have found for the most current and accurate information on Lp-(a) is Dr. Sinatra's website, his series of books, newsletters and more recently his blogs. He continues to study it and make recommendations accordingly. He has been a constant voice in the medical community raising awareness on this serious underemphasized problem. www.drsinatra.com

You've probably heard the joke; "Hey Doc it hurts when I do this?" And the doctor responds, "Well don't do that." Or the patient says, "Doc I'm much better, but I can't sing," and the doctor responds, "Could you sing before?" and the patient says, "Well no."It is with that philosophy I engage in exercise. I was never athletically inclined as a child, I'd trip going up a flight of stairs and when I ran I'd often kick my own rear end, literally. At the end of the school year they'd have what they called field days; where you'd run races, distance jumping and throwing. The teachers would look for a way for each child to achieve some form of a ribbon, not me. I received a certificate of attendance.

So I can't say that the heart attack really changed my tendency towards gentle simple exercise. However, it did refocus me on the importance of daily exercise. I excel in (easy) Therapeutic Yoga, Tai Chi, swimming and walking preferably outdoors. I don't like, or feel safe on a treadmill. I use my stationary bike on days that I don't want to exercise at all because I can watch TV and be distracted by my lazy mood. Sometimes I'll turn on an oldies radio station and just dance around the kitchen. After 10-15 minutes with any of these activities I can usually generate a decent sweat. Most days I exercise for 40 minutes then follow with meditation, but if I only have 30 minutes I no longer brow beat myself, the goal is consistency and that was difficult enough for me to achieve. Variety is important to keep me inspired. I have witnessed my energy noticeably decline if I don't exercise for few days. I need exercise for energy.

I love the beach. One of my favorite stops along the ocean boardwalk is the candy store where I purchase dark chocolate covered caramels. I allow myself only a quarter of a pound and tell myself that that will suffice my weekend trip. Yeah, well, that's a delusion, there gone in a couple of hours. But, it's only 6 pieces of candy…small scrumptious candy… and oh… my, gosh, they're so good. What I don't under-stand is how a quarter pound of chocolate can over night, put five extra pounds on the hips. It's one of life's great mysteries.

Weight management is very important, but you won't get any advice from me, I've struggled with my weight since I was in my mid thirties. I've tried all the diets. I swear I can gain weight just watching the food channels. My metabolism retired about twenty years ago. One of the first things my granddaughter learned from me as a toddler; was how to scream when she jumped on the scale.

My dad carried too much weight. My mom was very thin. My maternal grandparents were heavy. Is there a genetic component to weight or is it strictly environmental behaviors? I don't know, what I do know is; the older I get the more aches and pains I have, and I would like to weigh less. It's a source of frustration and stress. It is a high priority goal as much as I joke about it. Honestly, I prepare all my food with fresh ingredients, there no hidden sugars, high fructose corn syrup, salt, or partially hydrogenated fats; I know what I'm eating. I eat small quantities of lean meat. Mostly I use meat as a seasoning; for soups and stews. I consume a very Mediterranean diet.

Like finding a needle in a haystack, when I move again, I want to find a doctor that specializes in Integrative Medicine and that has a personal weight problem...

Notes from my heart:

What I know for sure, ten years later: It is a joint effort. You must address the needs of the spiritual heart to heal the physical heart.

1. You'll need to get real with yourself. Cut through the layers of responsibility and reach your raw emotions. Are your daily efforts expressing the authentic you. Are you forced by your circumstance to accept a steady diet of things that make you unhappy?

2. You need to give voice to your repressed emotions, through journaling, talk therapy, art therapy, a friendship or prayer.

3. What goes on behind your smile? What do you day dream about? When you identify your true passion, find ways to include it in daily life. Believe you will. If you don't expect it you won't get much.

4. Set goals to make the necessary changes; expect that there might be a realistic time delay in the transition. In the meantime remind yourself that it's temporary.

5. Adjust your perception; accept that you might have to be selfish at times for self-care.

6. Have mentors seek wisdom. The goal is an open heart.

7. Stay informed the resources for Alternative Care are better than ever. See my resource page.

8. I don't believe you are ever too busy doing the things you love or enjoy. The key is to find a balance between joy and necessity.

9. Recent studies have shown the importance of proper rest. You need seven to eight hours of sleep a night for health and well being.

Chapter 13:
The Soul

"The soul of Jonathan was knit to the soul of David and Jonathan loved him as himself." —1 Samuel 18:1

It happened purely by accident. My daughter was trying to take a picture of me as I turned to kiss (at that time) my youngest grandson. The picture captured the tender and precious love between us. It is an undeniable depiction of the child's acceptance of you and their need for your affection. As my lips caressed his baby flesh you could see his spirit melting into mine, and the bond begins. These are my most cherished possessions, what I call "kiss pictures." I have posed many times with our grandchildren, but by far, the special pictures are in their reaction to a kiss; as their natural spirit is exposed, so to, is their soul. For me, a student of the heart, I'm in constant search of the feel good moments that replenish my soul. These pictures provide that for me. My home is filled with collages that I've made over a thirty year period. With our ever growing family and numerous moves it allowed me a way to display life's moments and record the journey along the way. I'm always surrounded by our life's celebrated moments. While it started out as a hobby, over the years it became a form of therapy as well when I'd lose a loved one. It was my attempt to keep their presence in daily life.

Therapy released many buried memories. Of not only things I might have done differently. It also reminded me I lived each day with the purpose of providing or improving the lives of those around me. Like the "kiss pictures" I often self medicated with positive measures, that I performed or created. Although I was guilty of self neglect. On a daily basis I also committed acts of self love. Maybe that was the energy that sustained that barely open artery for so long.

Remember my original discussion with the Naturopath Director of the Complementary Care Clinic that suggested I was suffering from a broken heart? Of course I was. But when he connected that, to the heart attack and stents, he cast a different light on the same problem. I knew he was correct. The healing process of such has never been defined, except to say time will heal all wounds. No prescription…

I envisioned before I completed psychotherapy I would be able to place names or label each stent. I thought each stent represented a different heart ache or heart break. Stent #1 watching my Dad die of cancer…Stent #2…etc. That is not how it unfolded for me. It was a short time after I decided to end all therapies. I had been praying for guidance or approval that my decision was correct… And then I had a dream.

From my Roman Catholic upbringing I learned to meditate on the Rosary at an early age. When you need special consideration or favor, you pray your Rosary to the Virgin Mary as your intercessor to God. When you commit to a series of Rosary's over a period of days it's called a Novena. This practice of reciting the Rosary, I believe, has brought me closer to God. It has always been a great comfort to me to have this devotion to my Spiritual Mother. In prayer I could tell her the things I wanted to share with my own mother but never could, especially the despair I felt over the possibility of leaving my own children.

In my dream the Virgin Mary held me in her arms as she held her son. When I woke I remembered the vision vividly. A wonderful sensation of peace and gratitude enveloped me. I knew I was healed. In my moment of Glory I oddly heard a replay of my own voice from a few years earlier. Describing to my family the pain and anguish I experienced the night Kim died. "It was as though she was torn from my soul." I said, repeatedly, to anyone that would listen, trying to make sense of the pain. I went on and described in detail; "If I close my eyes and visualize my soul I can see it. My soul is inside my heart. And it's badly torn with jagged edges."

One of the get well gifts I received after I had my heart attack was a book titled, *"The Seat of the Soul"* by Gary Zukav. During my recovery I attempted many times to read the book but couldn't focus. I really wanted to read his book, I was drawn to it. Instead I used the book to measure my own ability to concentrate. Periodically I'd attempt it again and after a few minutes say, "okay not there yet, I'll try again next month." Possibly the book would have provided the soul insight that I needed. I struggled with some of my thoughts. I needed confirmation that others had similar experiences. When I read the Ancient Greeks believed that your soul resides in your heart. It stimulated an out loud-Alleluia!

The remedy was waiting for me. Just as I started to write this book, *"The Seat of the Soul"* by Gary Zukav fell off my book shelf, still unread after ten years. I couldn't put it down; I read it in a day. It had a profound effect on me. The book is a beautifully written journey that takes you past the five senses. There were a few sentences from his book that tied together my final thoughts of that difficult period of my life. The first is his description of psychology: *"Psychology means soul knowledge."* And the subsequent is defined in his chapter about, *The Soul.* He writes; *"The body needs rest and it needs care, but behind every aspect of the health or illness of the body is the energy of the soul. It is the health of the soul that is the true purpose of the human experience."*

My traumatic human experience brought me to soul school of sorts, through the two years of psychotherapy. The combined effort of pampering my body, and the soul search was necessary to restore me. I said from the introduction there's no one size cure all on disease. But for me, someone that resides in my sixth sense, the additional efforts were mandatory. It is my belief the seven stents represent what was once my shattered soul; each stent has sewn together and mended the jagged edges. Through the restoration of my soul, my heart was healed.

While I had soul ties to all my family that had past, with Kim it was different. I also felt responsible. When she was born I was three years old, my brother was two years old, and my mom had a miscarriage between and after their births. For years my mom was always pregnant and always sick. My older sisters were already school age, when I became mom's very little helper. It was always; "watch your sister, keep an eye on your brother," and as they got older it unnaturally progressed in my mom's mind that anything they did wrong had

136

to be my fault. As a teenager I rebelled at her logic, but deep inside my soul I never let go of the responsibility. There was definitely a confusion of roles, and when Kim died I asked myself how I could let this happen to her. In my hysteria it was my fault, I should have protected her. For two years in therapy Kim was the 400 pound gorilla in the room. I refused to discuss her, other than at one point I admitted to my therapist I had a survivor's guilt. Not everything could be resolved in therapy; some things were between me and God. Eventually I graduated from the unreasonable responsibilities placed on me and I found forgiveness. It was five years after the death of my sister and three years after my heart attack, through a shattered soul, to heart break... I returned to wholeness.

My life has been a series of surrenders and then, release. The spirit of that house, my healing place was releasing me. I was healed, and there was a new journey just around the corner. Me and my big mouth declaring, "Death is not an option, I have too much to do." God held me to my words.

And then the Angels started to tickle me... "Chicago! I don't want to move back to Chicago! Our kids and grandchildren are on the East Coast!" The events of 9/11 seriously affected the hotel industry and the downsizing began at the top. My husband was very fortunate to have a job offer as quickly as he did, actually he had two. One would have taken us to Texas-a foreign land to me, the other was a terrific position in Chicago. He wore me down with; "I'm tired of all the traveling and this position would allow me to be home more." Red flag...Red flag..."I'm tired," he had never complained before. I immediately agreed. Of course as I put the house on the market to sell; the pipes cracked, the roof sprung a leak and our dog gave birth to twelve puppies...

Notes from my heart:

What I know for sure, ten years later. My passage has encouraged a deeper connection to my soul, with love as my spiritual guide. The following are ideas for replenishing the soul, this may be the first ever prescription for healing a broken heart. Maybe we should just call it, "My Recipe."

1. Try meditation, if you find setting aside time difficult, begin small. Start with two minutes at the same time each day.

2. As you increase your meditation time you will connect with your inner self and begin to hear your inner voice.

3. Learning breathing techniques are very important they can lower blood pressure quickly and the breaths will calm you. I use it as a trigger when I'm upset about something. I simply say to myself; "calm down and breathe. I then take three slow deep breaths.

4. Develop better habits; take mental health breaks throughout the day: Mini retreats. Even 10 to 20 minutes is enough. Listen to soothing music or guided imagery.

5. More soul medicine? Do you love the beach or hiking? If you can't afford a trip to the ocean, don't wait, maybe a nearby lake would suffice; sun, water, sand and birds. Every state and most towns have hiking trails.

6. With a little imagination you can create your own free retreat in your home or nearby.

7. Make a commitment to take time every day for self-care and soul replenishment, whether ten minutes or an hour long, mini-retreats have restorative power.

8. Some of my favorites: Relax in a bath with fragrant oil or bubbles, soft music or a relaxation CD.

9. Go for a walk and open your senses to the beauty of the world.

10. Ten minutes on a massage chair or foot massager is perfect.

11. I take power naps-20 minutes and I'm good for hours.

12. Take a ten minute dance break to your favorite beat.

13. Combine a passion with a disliked chore. I listen to opera when I need to clean out a closet. I restore order and replenish my soul at the same time.

14. Restorative yoga is one of the gentlest styles of yoga. You will be taken through a series of poses that will aid digestion, promote relaxation and restore the vitality of your body and mind. Class begins and closes with guided meditation and yogic breathing techniques that will de-stress your body and calm your mind.

15. Read to a child or read for yourself.

16. Laughter... more laughter.

17. Oh the power of prayer.

18. Take care of all your senses. Eat a favorite food at least once a week.

19. Surround yourself with the things that are beautiful to you.

20. Do what you love.

Chapter 14:
Celebrating Love

"Being deeply loved by someone gives you strength, while loving someone deeply gives you courage." —Lao Tzu

When I was a child my birthday present was a little, brown, bag filled with penny candy. The party was sharing with my siblings, and counting the candies in the bag. It seemed like a million. No candles required. We'd just giggle from our sugar high and sing happy birthday. My Dad never let us down and you could bet he'd come home from work earlier in anticipation. It was our special day. It was simple. It was fun. And we knew we were loved.

While I've turned family celebrations into an art form, I'm mindful of the intention; to remind that person how much they are loved and adored. On your special day, you chose your favorite meal, complete with dessert. Birthday presents are bought per your specifications because it's important to me that you know I'm listening. I perfected these celebrations, during my; "Hurricane in Heels" years. It was my cover-up, for anything I might have missed or screwed up throughout the year. You should see our Christmas Eve celebration; I literally start planning it after Halloween.

Bill Cosby tells a joke about his parents, it goes something like this: "These are not the same people that raised me these are old people that are trying to get into heaven."

There's comes a time in life when your more concerned about your legacy of memories. This awareness probably occurred to me sooner than most because of my circumstances. So that becomes a goal; creating the best possible moments.

Last year my mom and mother-in-law died two months apart. As they transitioned I studied their behavior. Both women were in poor health. However, I viewed their spirits sustain them until they achieved their personal objectives. At 93 years old, after receiving four last rites and two separate tours of hospice care, my mother-in-law survived to be at our daughter's wedding. Though she was legally blind, wheel chair bound racked with pain from osteoarthritis, osteoporosis and near deaf, I watched and listened as she recited the Lord's Prayer at the wedding. After the wedding she stopped eating again and past a few weeks later.

When Kim died our mom shared responsibility with my brother-in-law and raised their three children. I was never more proud of her. She would remind me they were her reason to get up every morning. Mom wasn't well all winter and continued to lose weight, everyone tried to get her to see a doctor. She said it was the stomach flu. By late May her granddaughter graduated from college and her grandson graduated from high school. It was no coincidence to me that my Mom lived to see both. I spent her last days with her. While she didn't elaborate, as was her style, she simply said to me, "I'm done now Pam." My Mom died two weeks after their graduations. How fortunate I was to have these two women of purpose in my life, and experience the lessons of their spirits.

Having witnessed the long goodbyes as in Dementia and Alzheimer's, to the more average length of goodbye due to terminal cancer, to the instant death with heart disease-I've come to terms or acceptance. Where I couldn't imagine at the time of loss that I'd ever understand the purpose-my walk with God has blessed me with an "insight." Their existence graced our lives; they were our gift. And for those, whose time is cut short, their deaths promoted change, whether it was a change in habits, or the lifestyle of others. Their death reminded us how precious life is. Now they are our Angels.

Maybe sometimes death is about a greater good. Just as science suggests women are protected from heart disease until menopause, I think when we observe a mother with three young children; we naturally want to believe that there is a protective umbrella around her to raise those children. But, who is the better teacher? It's those deaths that make us gasp for air when we hear about them, that we are most impacted by.

Remember my mantra? I have prophesized, "living well, past eighty five." That should suffice the current promises I've made to my older grandchildren; that I'll be there when they graduate from medical school. And dance a polka at their wedding. Yeah, they cringe at that thought. There's no need to hire an accordion player just yet. What they don't know is, I can't skip or jump, so I don't polka either. But baby, I can twist! Maybe we'll just let their grandfather lead us in a mellow Greek Dance.

Anyway I have about thirty more years. If that's not enough time for all my future appointments and celebrations, not to worry, I'll negotiate for more time. I always have my secret weapon; the row boat and Novena's. In the meantime I've committed every waking moment of my journey, to love. To me, the greatest tragedy would be to leave the world with things unsaid.

Epilogue

Just pace yourself, breathe and try to enjoy the new journey. You're in control, you're not alone. Oh God all those years that I wished to move my family home to Chicago why now when it is the least of my desires. But like so many times before, I was forced to surrender.

It was a mid September morning, 2003. We were welcomed home by my brother's smile and a chilly 34 degree temperature as we pulled into the driveway of our new home in a Chicago suburb.

By Christmas Night that year I understood the purpose behind our move. As we went to bed that night Chris screamed, a horrible, pain filled, scream. He was experiencing a large brain hemorrhage from a malformation in his brain, a form of a stroke. We found out later that he was born with it. As it was told to me if you're lucky, you'll develop headaches in your twenties and hopefully it's found. If not, the arterial venous malformation of the brain will likely burst in your fifties. His hemorrhage was on time; that September he had turned 51, and he had an appointment with destiny.

Although the ambulance arrived with minutes, time went downhill immediately. After hours of wasted time at our local hospital he was accepted by and transported via helicopter to The University of Chicago Hospital. He miraculously survived the ordeal. The neuro-team nick named him, "The Miracle Man," that Christmas week. He was well past the window of opportunity for improved outcomes. "Time lost is brain lost," was The American Stroke Association slogan at the time. He spent weeks in a coma and years in therapy. He needed five years of full-time care to undo the damage caused in those lost hours. To this day his brain is still regenerating and connecting bridges around the injured areas.

As I said, the moves we made were meant to be. There were people we were meant to meet along the way. This time my husband would receive surgery from a brilliant Neurosurgeon that specialized in, and wrote the procedure for a ruptured AVM: arterial venous malformation of the brain. It was where we needed to be that Christmas Night, in Chicago.

Important Resources:

Medical Doctors that also specialize in Complementary/Integrative Care:
- Dr. Stephen Sinatra-www.drsinatra .com
- Dr. Andrew Weil-www.drweil.com
- Dr. Mehmet Oz-www.doctoroz.com
- Dr. Christiane Northrup-drnorthrup.com
-

Guided Imagery, Breath work, Meditation, Yoga, Acupressure, Tai Chi and Aromatherapy:
- Belleruth Naparstak –www.Healthjourneys.com
-

Yoga:
- Peggy Cappy: www.peggycappy.com

www.ingramcontent.com/pod-product-compliance
Lightning Source LLC
Chambersburg PA
CBHW032002190326
41520CB00007B/325